Denying to the Grave

Denying
to the Grave

Why We Ignore the Facts
That Will Save Us

SARA E. GORMAN, PhD, MPH

JACK M. GORMAN, MD

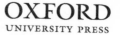

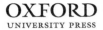
OXFORD
UNIVERSITY PRESS

Oxford University Press is a department of the University of Oxford. It furthers
the University's objective of excellence in research, scholarship, and education
by publishing worldwide. Oxford is a registered trade mark of Oxford University
Press in the UK and certain other countries.

Published in the United States of America by Oxford University Press
198 Madison Avenue, New York, NY 10016, United States of America.

© Oxford University Press 2017

A copy of this book's Cataloging-in-Publication Data is on file with the Library of Congress.

ISBN 978-0-19-939660-3

9 8 7 6 5 4 3 2 1

Printed by Sheridan Books, Inc., United States of America

Authors' Note
The information in this book is not intended to replace the advice of the reader's own
physician or other medical professional. You should consult a medical professional in
matters relating to your health, especially if you have existing medical conditions, and
before starting, stopping or changing the dose of any medication you are taking. Individual
readers are solely responsible for their own health care decisions. The author and the
publisher do not accept responsibility for any adverse effects individuals may claim to
experience, whether directly or indirectly, from the information contained in this book.

In memory of Howard Kantor, tireless devotee of science and medicine, beloved father, grandfather, and husband

Contents

Acknowledgments

We would like to express our gratitude to all the wonderful, inspiring people who helped us write this book. First and foremost, we thank all of the brilliant scholars and medical and public health practitioners, without whose contributions to our growing body of knowledge about neuroscience, psychology, and health decision making this book would have been impossible to write. We'd like to thank in particular the following scholars, who all generously served as interlocutors at some stage during the writing of this book: Daniel Kahneman, Michael Shermer, Seth Mnookin, Tal Gross, and Nicoli Nattrass. We are very grateful to the anonymous reviewers of the book whose input was critical in shaping and improving our final product. We are indebted to the wonderful people at Oxford University Press, including Andrea Zekus, who helped us along this sometimes arduous process, and of course, our fantastic editor, Sarah Harrington, whose sharp insight was always much appreciated.

Sara would also like to thank her colleagues and mentors at work for allowing her the time and flexibility to work on the book and for supporting and encouraging her along the way. She's also extremely grateful to Wendy Olesker for all her support.

Many people provided intellectual and emotional support to Jack that was indispensable in writing this book, and he is especially grateful to Robert Wainwright, Richard Munich, Catherine DiDesidero, Bruce Brady, Rabbi Avi Weiss, Alexandra Roth-Kahn, Stan Arkow, Marc Suvall, Carol Clayton, Leigh Steiner, and David Bressman for their creative ideas and friendship.

Finally, there are many amazing people in our personal lives who have offered us critical support as we undertook this journey. Because we are father and daughter, we have most of them in common. We are deeply grateful to Rachel Moster, Sara's sister and Jack's daughter, and David Moster, Rachel's husband, for being our all-time champions, for always being there for us, and for always sharing our excitement with their overwhelming warmth, intellectual prowess, and zest.

Two people are the bedrock and inspiration for all we do. Lauren Kantor Gorman, Sara's mother and Jack's wife, is the beacon of light in the madness that sometimes comes from writing a book. As a brilliant psychiatrist, she has wonderful insights into the emotional basis for people's choices and decisions that helped us enormously in focusing our own ideas. We thank her for always being so steady, reliable, and smart, and for showering us with her constant love and warmth. Last but by no means least, we'd like to thank Robert Kohen, Sara's husband and Jack's son-in-law. Robert is our brilliant interlocutor, our intellectual companion, and our unending inspiration. Thank you for being you.

Denying to the Grave

Introduction

ON OCTOBER 8, 2014, THOMAS ERIC DUNCAN DIED IN A Dallas hospital from Ebola virus infection. From the moment he was diagnosed with Ebola newspapers all over the country blared the news that the first case of Ebola in the United States had occurred. Blame for his death was immediately assigned to the hospital that cared for him and to the U.S. Centers for Disease Control and Prevention (CDC).[1] By the end of the month a total of four cases had developed in the United States: two in people—including Duncan—who acquired it in African countries where the disease was epidemic and two in nurses who cared for Duncan. Headlines about Ebola continued to dominate the pages of American newspapers throughout the month, warning of the risk we now faced of this deadly disease. These media reports were frightening and caused some people to wonder if it was safe to send their children to school or ride on public transportation—even if they lived miles from any of the four cases. "There are reports of kids being pulled out of schools and even some school closings," reported Dean Baker in the *Huffington Post*. "People in many areas are not going to work and others are driving cars rather than taking mass transit because they fear catching Ebola from fellow passengers. There are also reports of people staying away from stores, restaurants, and other public places."[2] An elementary school in Maine suspended a teacher because she stayed in a hotel in Dallas that is 9.5 miles away from the hospital where two nurses contracted the virus.[3] As Charles Blow put it in his *New York Times* column, "We aren't battling a virus in this country as much as a mania, one whipped up by reactionary politicians and irresponsible media."[4]

It turns out that Thomas Duncan was not the only person who died in the United States on October 8, 2014. If we extrapolate from national annual figures, we can say that on that day almost 7,000 people died in the United States. About half of them died of either heart disease or cancer; 331 from accidents, of which automobile accidents are the most common; and 105 by suicide.[5] About 80 people were killed by gunshot wounds the day that Thomas Eric Duncan died, two thirds of which were self-inflicted. NPR correspondent Michaeleen Doucleff made a rough calculation and determined that the risk of contracting Ebola in the United States was 1 in 13.3 million, far less than the risk of dying in a plane crash, from a bee sting, by being struck by lightning, or being attacked by a shark.[6] The chance of being killed in a car crash is about 1,500 times greater than the risk of getting infected with the Ebola virus in the United States.

It probably comes as no surprise that there were very few front-page headlines about bee stings or shark attacks on October 8, 2014, let alone about car crashes and gun violence. Perhaps this seems natural. After all, Ebola virus infection, the cause of Ebola hemorrhagic fever (EHF), is unusual in the United States, whereas heart attacks, cancer, car crashes, suicide, and murder happen on a regular basis. The problem, however, with the media emphasizing (and ordinary people fearing) Ebola over other far more prevalent health threats is that it shapes our behavior, sometimes in dangerous ways. How many people smoked a cigarette or consumed a sugary breakfast cereal while reading about the threat they faced in catching Ebola?

Some Americans jumped on the blame game bandwagon, attacking the CDC, insisting that politicians and hospitals had dropped the ball, and accusing African countries of ignorant, superstitious behavior. In Washington, DC, one-quarter of the members of Trinity Episcopal Church stopped attending services because they feared that some fellow parishioners might have traveled to West Africa.[7] An Ohio bridal shop owner reported losing tens of thousands of dollars because Amber Vinson, one of two Dallas-based nurses who tested positive for Ebola, had visited her shop. The owner closed the store during the incubation period and had the store profession-ally cleaned, but "a string of frightened customers cancelled their orders."[8] According to a presidential commission report, "Americans focused on their own almost nonexistent risk of catching Ebola from travelers instead of pressing to help the truly affected nations."[9] It is quite likely that most of these frightened Americans did not increase their exercise, cut down on eating processed foods, fasten their seat belts, quit smoking, make sure guns in the home were unloaded in locked cases, or get help for depression and alcoholism. The novelty of Ebola was exciting, like watching a horror movie. Those other causes of death are familiar and boring. In other words, Americans acted in an irrational way, overestimating the risk of Ebola and underestimating the risk of the life-threatening phenomena about which they might be able to do something. As Sara pointed out in an article she wrote that month, "What is the most effective treatment for Americans to protect themselves from early death by an infec-tious pathogen? A flu shot."[10]

Fear of Ebola "gripped the country" after Dr. Craig Spencer was diagnosed with Ebola and was admitted to New York City's Bellevue Hospital.[11] Comparing this dramatic fear about something that is not a real health threat—Ebola infection in the United States—to the more muted concern about things that really threaten our health—lack of exercise, smoking, eating sugary foods, drinking too much alcohol, not wearing seat belts, owning guns—illustrates our per-sistent failure to use scientific evidence in making decisions about what we do to maintain and improve our health and our lives. This drives scientists, healthcare experts, and public health officials nuts. When an educated parent refuses to vaccinate her child because she fears the vaccination will do more harm than good, these experts decry the "ignorance" of that stance and cite the reams of evidence that prove the contrary is the case. Time after time, we make deci-sions about the health of ourselves and our families based on emo-tion rather than on analysis of the scientific data. The government uses taxpayer money to mount hugely expensive studies in order to prove that the science is correct, but people come up with more and more reasons to insist that the research is incomplete, biased, or simply wrong. Opposing camps accuse each other of deliberately plotting to harm the American public, of being bought off by special interests, and of stupidity. The data may be clear about who is right and who is wrong, but people make decisions that ignore or deny the evidence. This book is an attempt to elucidate why we do this and what we can do to make better decisions about our health and the health of our loved ones.

Why Do We Ignore or Deny Scientific Evidence?

It turns out that there are many reasons for refusing to acknowledge scientific evidence when making health decisions, but stupidity is not one of them. Very smart people take positions that are not remotely based on evidence. There is a direct relationship, for example, between intelligence and refusing to vaccinate a child: this unfortunate behavior is championed mainly by very well-educated and affluent people.[12] What then causes smart people to make decisions and adopt positions that have no factual basis? That is the question with which this book wrestles.

The idea for this book took shape as Sara became increasingly involved in the world of public health. She was particularly mystified by the "anti-vaxxers," people who promulgate the notion that immunizations are harmful, causing, among other things, autism. Nothing could be further from the truth. Immunization is one of the triumphs of modern medicine, having eliminated from our lives deadly diseases such as smallpox, measles, polio, and diphtheria. It is based on elegant scientific principles, has a remarkable safety record, and absolutely does not cause autism. How could anyone, Sara wondered, refuse to vaccinate a child?

At the same time Jack, who trained as a psychiatrist and worked as a scientist most of his career, was increasingly interested in the reasons people own guns. He thought at first it was for hunting and decided that just because it was a hobby that neither he nor any of his New York City friends pursued, it would be wrong to advocate that all the people who enjoy shooting animals in the woods be prevented from doing so. But a look at the data showed that a relatively small number of Americans are hunters and that most gun owners have weapons for "protection." Yet studies show over and over again that a gun in the house is far more likely to be used to injure or kill someone who lives there than to kill an intruder. Gun availability is clearly linked to elevated risk for both homicide and suicide.[13] Statistically speaking, the risks of having a gun at home are far greater than any possible benefits. Consider the tragic case of 26-year-old St. Louis resident Becca Campbell, who bought a gun reportedly to protect herself and her two daughters. Instead of protecting herself and her family from risks such as the Ferguson riots, she wound up accidentally shooting and killing herself with it.[14]

In both cases scientific evidence strongly suggests a position—vaccinate your child and don't keep a gun at home—that many of us choose to ignore or deny. We make a distinction between "ignore" and "deny," the former indicating that a person does not know the scientific evidence and the latter that he or she does but actively disagrees with it. We quickly generated a list of several other health and healthcare beliefs that fly directly in the face of scientific evidence and that are supported by at least a substantial minority of people:

- Vaccination is harmful.
- Guns in the house will protect residents from armed intruders.
- Foods containing genetically modified organisms (GMOs) are dangerous to human health.
- The human immunodeficiency virus (HIV) is not the cause of AIDS.
- Nuclear power is more dangerous than power derived from burning fossil fuels.
- Antibiotics are effective in treating viral infections.
- Unpasteurized milk is safe and contains beneficial nutrients that are destroyed by the pasteurization process.
- Electroconvulsive therapy (ECT, or shock treatment) causes brain damage and is ineffective.

Throughout this book we present evidence that none of these positions is correct. But our aim is not to exhaustively analyze scientific data and studies. Many other sources review in rigorous detail the evidence that counters each of these eight beliefs. Rather, our task is to try to understand *why* reasonably intelligent and well-meaning people believe them.

Many of the thought processes that allow us to be human, to have empathy, to function in society, and to survive as a species from an evolutionary standpoint can lead us astray when applied to what scientists refer to as *scientific reasoning*. Why? For starters, scientific reasoning is difficult for many people to accept because it precludes the ability to make positive statements with certainty. Scientific reasoning, rather, works by setting up hypotheses to be knocked down, makes great demands before causality can be demonstrated, and involves populations instead of individuals. In other words, in science we can never be 100% sure. We can only be very close to totally sure. This runs counter to the ways we humans are accustomed to thinking. Moreover, science works through a series of negations and disproving, while we are wired to resist changing our minds too easily. As a result, a multitude of completely healthy and normal psychological processes can conspire to make us prone to errors in scientific and medical thinking, leading to decisions that adversely affect our health.

These poor health decisions often involve adopting risky behaviors, including refusal to be vaccinated, consumption of unhealthy food, cigarette smoking, failure to adhere to a medication regimen, and failure to practice safe sex. We believe that these risk-taking behaviors stem in large part from complex psychological factors that often have known biological underpinnings. In this book we explore the psychology and neurobiology of poor health decisions and irrational health beliefs, arguing that in many cases the psychological impulses under discussion are *adaptive* (meaning, they evolved to keep us safe and healthy), but are often applied in a *maladaptive* way. We also argue that without proper knowledge of the psychological and biological underpinnings of irrational health decisions and beliefs, we as a society cannot design any strategy that will alleviate the problem. We therefore conclude by offering our own method of combatting poor health decision making, a method that takes into account psychology and neurobiology and that offers guidance on how to encourage people to adopt a more scientific viewpoint without discounting or trying to eliminate their valuable emotional responses.

We will assert many times that the problem is not simply lack of information, although that can be a factor. Irrational behavior occurs even when we know and understand all the facts. Given what we now understand about brain function, it is probably not even appropriate to label science denial as, strictly speaking, "irrational." Rather, it is for the most part a product of the way our minds work. This means that simple education is not going to be sufficient to reverse science denial. Certainly, angry harangues at the "stupidity" of science denialists will only reify these attitudes. Take, for example, a recent article in *The Atlantic* that discussed affluent Los Angeles parents who refuse to have their children vaccinated, concluding, "Wealth enables these people to hire fringe pediatricians who will coddle their irrational beliefs. But it doesn't entitle them to threaten an entire city's children with terrifying, 19th-century diseases for no reason."[15] This stance is unhelpful because it attempts to shame people into changing their beliefs and behaviors, a strategy that rarely works when it comes to health and medicine. As Canadian scientists Chantal Pouliot and Julie Godbout point out in their excellent article on public science education, when scientists think about communicating with nonscientists, they generally operate from the "knowledge deficit" model, the idea that nonscientists simply lack the facts. Evidence shows, these authors argue instead, that nonscientists are in fact capable of understanding "both the complexity of research and the uncertainties accompanying many technological and scientific developments."[16] Pouliot and Godbout call for educating scientists about social scientists' research findings that show the public is indeed capable of grasping scientific concepts.

Each of the six chapters of this book examines a single key driver of science denial. Each one of them rests on a combination of psychological, behavioral, sociological, political, and neurobiological components. We do not insist that these are the only reasons for science denial, but through our own work and research we have come to believe that they are among the most important and the most prominent.

Just Because You're Paranoid Doesn't Mean People Aren't Conspiring Against You

In chapter 1, "Conspiracy Theories," we address the complicated topic of conspiracy theories. Complicated because a conspiracy theory is not *prima facie* wrong and indeed there have been many conspiracies that we would have been better off uncovering when they first occurred. Yet one of the hallmarks of false scientific beliefs is the claim by their adherents that they are the victims of profiteering, deceit, and cover-ups by conglomerates variously composed of large corporations, government regulatory agencies, the media, and professional medical societies. The trick is to figure out if the false ones can be readily separated from those in which there may be some truth.

Only by carefully analyzing a number of such conspiracy theories and their adherents does it become possible to offer some guidelines as to which are most obviously incorrect. More important for our purposes, we explore the psychology of conspiracy theory adherence. What do people get out of believing in false conspiracy theories? How does membership in a group of like-minded conspiracy theorists develop, and why is it so hard to persuade people that they are wrong? As is the case with every reason we give in this book for adherence to false scientific ideas, belittling people who come to believe in false conspiracy theories as ignorant or mean-spirited is perhaps the surest route to reinforcing an anti-science position.

Charismatic Leaders

Perhaps the biggest and most formidable opponents to rational understanding and acceptance of scientific evidence in the health field are what are known as charismatic leaders, our second factor in promoting science denial. In chapter 2, "Charismatic Leaders," we give several profiles of leaders of anti-science movements and try to locate common denominators among them. We stress that most people who hold incorrect ideas about health and deny scientific evidence are well-meaning individuals who believe that they are doing the right thing for themselves and their families. We also stress that the very same mental mechanisms that we use to generate incorrect ideas about scientific issues often have an evolutionary basis, can be helpful and healthy in many circumstances, and may even make us empathic individuals.

When we deal with charismatic figures, however, we are often dealing with people for whom it is difficult to generate kind words. Although they may be true believers, most of them are people who should know better, who often distort the truth, and who may masquerade as selfless but in fact gain considerable personal benefit from promulgating false ideas. And, most important, what they do harms people.

There is a fascinating, albeit at times a bit frightening, psychology behind the appeal of these charismatic leaders that may help us be more successful in neutralizing their hold over others. Although many of them have impressive-sounding academic credentials, the factors that can make them seem believable may be as trivial as having a deep voice.[17] Chapter 2 marks the end of a two-chapter focus on the psychology of groups and how it fosters anti-science beliefs.

If I Thought It Once, It Must Be True

Everyone looks for patterns in the environment. Once we find them and if they seem to explain things we become more and more convinced we need them. The ancients who thought the sun revolved around the earth were not stupid, nor were they entirely ruled by religious dogma that humans must be at the center of the earth. In fact, if you look up in the sky, that is at first what seems to be happening. After years of observation and calculation, the Greek astronomer Ptolemy devised a complicated mathematical system to explain the rotation of stars around the earth. It is not a simple explanation but rather the work of a brilliant mind using all of the tools available to him. Of course, it happens to be wrong. But once it was written down and taught to other astronomers it became hard to give up. Rather, as new observations came in that may have challenged the "geocentric" model, astronomers were apt to do everything possible to fit them into the "earth as the center of the universe" idea. That is, they saw what they believed.

It took another set of geniuses—Copernicus, Kepler, and Galileo—and new inventions like the telescope to finally dislodge the Ptolemaic model.

Once any such belief system is in place, it becomes the beneficiary of what is known as the confirmation bias. Paul Slovic captured the essence of confirmation bias, the subject of chapter 3, very well:

> It would be comforting to believe that polarized positions would respond to informational and educational programs. Unfortunately, psychological research demonstrates that people's beliefs change slowly and are extraordinarily persistent in the face of contrary evidence (Nisbett & Ross, 1980). Once formed, initial impressions tend to structure the way that subsequent evidence is interpreted. New evidence appears reliable and informative if it is consistent with one's initial beliefs; contrary evidence is dismissed as unreliable, erroneous or unrepresentative.[18]

Does this sound familiar? We can probably all think of examples in our lives in which we saw things the way we believed they should be rather than as they really were. For many years, for example, Jack believed that antidepressant medications were superior to cognitive behavioral therapy (CBT) in the treatment of an anxiety condition called panic disorder. That is what his professors insisted was true and it was part of being an obedient student to believe them. When studies were published that showed that CBT worked, he searched hard for flaws in the experimental methods or interpretation of those studies in order to convince himself that the new findings were not sufficient to dislodge his belief in medication's superiority. Finally, he challenged a CBT expert, David Barlow, now of Boston University, to do a study comparing the two forms of treatment and, to his surprise, CBT worked better than medication.[19]

Fortunately, Jack let the data have its way and changed his mind, but until that point he worked hard to confirm his prior beliefs. This happens all the time in science and is the source of some very passionate scientific debates and conflicts in every field. It also turns out that neuroscientists, using sophisticated brain imaging techniques, have been able to show the ways in which different parts of the brain respond to challenges to fixed ideas with either bias or open-mindedness. The challenge for those of us who favor adherence to scientific evidence is to support the latter. In this effort we are too often opposed by anti-science charismatic leaders.

If A Came Before B, Then A Caused B

Uncertainty, as we explain in chapter 4, "Causality and Filling the Ignorance Gap," is uncomfortable and even frightening to many people. It is a natural tendency to want to know why things are as they are, and this often entails figuring out what caused what. Once again, this tendency is almost certainly an evolutionarily conserved, protective feature—when you smell smoke in your cave you assume there is a fire causing it and run; you do not first consider alternative explanations or you might not survive. We are forced to assign causal significance to things we observe every day. If you hear the crash of a broken glass and see your dog running out of the room, you reach the conclusion immediately that your dog has knocked a glass off a tabletop. Of course, it is possible that something else knocked the glass off and frightened the dog into running, what epidemiologists might call reverse causation, but that would be an incorrect conclusion most of the time. Without the propensity to assign causality we would once again get bogged down in all kinds of useless considerations and lose our ability to act.

In many ways, however, the causality assumption will fail us when we are considering more complicated systems and issues. This is not a "chicken and egg" problem; that is a philosophical and linguistic conundrum that has no scientific significance. We know that chickens hatch from eggs and also lay eggs so that neither the chicken nor egg itself actually came first but rather evolutionarily more primitive life forms preceded both. By causality we are talking here instead about the way in which the scientific method permits us to conclude that something is the cause of something else. If you look again at our list of examples of anti-science views, you can see that a number of them are the result of disputes over causality. There is no question, for example, that HIV causes AIDS, and we are similarly certain that vaccines do not cause autism. Yet there are individuals and groups that dispute these clear scientific facts about causality.

If one has a child with autism the temptation to find a cause for it is perfectly understandable. The uncertainty of why a child has autism is undoubtedly part of the heartbreak faced by parents. Many initially blame themselves. Perhaps the mom should not have eaten so much fried food during pregnancy. Or maybe it is because the dad has a bad gene or was too old to father a child. Guilt sets in, adding to the anguish of having a child who will struggle throughout his or her life to fit in. Such parents in distress become highly prone to leap to a causality conclusion if one becomes available, especially if it allows us to be angry at someone else instead of ourselves. Once an idea like vaccines cause autism is circulated and supported by advocacy groups it becomes very hard for scientists to dislodge it by citing data from all the studies showing that the conclusion is wrong. So the tendency to want or need to find causal links will often lead us to incorrect or even dangerous scientific conclusions.

It's Complicated

What is it about Ebola that makes it an epidemic in some West African countries like Liberia, Guinea, and Sierra Leone but a very small threat in America? Why, on the other hand, is the flu virus a major threat to the health of Americans, responsible for thousands of deaths in the last 30 years? The answer lies in the biology of these viruses. The Ebola virus, like HIV and influenza, is an RNA virus that is converted to DNA once inside a human cell, which allows it to insert itself into the host cells' genome, to replicate and then move on to infect more host cells. Its main reservoir is the fruit bat. Most important, it is spread by contact with bodily fluids of an infected individual;[20] it is not, like flu or chicken pox, an airborne virus. This is a very important point: one can catch the flu from someone merely by sitting nearby and inhaling the air into which he or she coughs or sneezes. A person can infect another person with the flu from as far as six feet away. Ebola does not spread that way. One has to handle the blood, urine, feces, or vomit of someone with Ebola in order to get it. Hence, the chance of spreading flu is much greater than the chance of spreading Ebola. The people most at risk for contracting Ebola are healthcare workers and family members who care for infected people. The incubation period for the Ebola virus is between 2 and 21 days, and an individual is not contagious until he or she becomes symptomatic. This is also different from the flu, which can be spread a day before a person becomes symptomatic. Thus, we know when a person with Ebola is contagious; we may not if the person has the flu.

Did you get all of that? Those are the facts. Do you now understand the difference between RNA and DNA viruses or the mechanisms by which viruses infect cells and replicate, or even exactly what replication is? Is the difference between bodily fluids and airborne infection completely clear, and do you understand what we mean by incubation period? Don't be surprised if you don't. These terms are second nature to doctors and most scientists, but other educated people probably don't think about them very much. Just as most doctors do not understand what cost-based accounting entails, most accountants are not expert virologists. In other words, the details of what Ebola is and does are complicated. Despite the common refrain that we are in a new era of information brought on by the World Wide Web, our brains are still not programmed to welcome technical and complex descriptions. You may have read the paragraph before this one quickly and committed to memory only words like HIV, bats, infect, symptomatic, and spread. Thus, if you are like most people you can read that paragraph and walk away only thinking, incorrectly, that "Ebola is infectious and you can get it from another person sitting next to you on the train."

Chapter 5, "Avoidance of Complexity," deals with another reason people succumb to unscientific notions—the discomfort we all have with complexity. It isn't that we are incapable of learning the facts but rather we are reluctant to put in the time and effort to do so. This may especially be the case when science and math are involved because many people believe, often incorrectly, that they are incapable of understanding those disciplines except in their most basic aspects. As we explain when we discuss some aspects of brain function, our minds gravitate naturally to clear and simple explanations of things, especially when they are laced with emotional rhetoric. We are actually afraid of complexity. Our natural instinct is to try to get our arms around an issue quickly, not to "obsess" or get caught in the weeds about it. As we indicate throughout this book, this retreat from complexity is similar to the other reasons for science denial in that it is in many ways a useful and adaptive stance. We would be paralyzed if we insisted on understanding the technical details of everything in our lives. One need have very little idea about how a car engine works in order to get in and drive; music can be enjoyed without fully understanding the relationships among major and minor keys and the harmonics of stringed instruments; a garden can be planted without an ability to write down all the chemical steps involved in photosynthesis and plant oxygen exchange. Furthermore, when we have to make urgent decisions it is often best not to dwell on the details. Emergencies are best handled by people who can act, not deliberate.

But when making health decisions, the inability to tackle scientific details can leave us prone to accepting craftily packaged inaccuracies and slogans. Scientists, doctors, and public health experts are often not helpful in this regard because they frequently refuse to explain things clearly and interestingly. Scientists seem to waver between overly complicated explanations that only they can fathom and overly simplistic explanations that feel patronizing and convey minimal useful information. Experts are also prone to adhering to simplistic and incorrect ideas when the truth is complicated.

In fact, as we argue in chapter 5, scientists need to work much harder on figuring out the best ways to communicate facts to non-scientists. This must begin by changing the way we teach science to children, from one of pure memorization to an appreciation of the way science actually works. By focusing on the scientific method, we can begin to educate people about how to accept complexity and uncertainty, how to be skeptical, and how to ask the right questions.

Who's Afraid of the Shower?

Chapter 6, "Risk Perception and Probability," focuses on something that is highlighted by the puzzle described in the opening passages of this book, about Ebola virus infection: an inability to appreciate true risk. The chance of getting Ebola virus in America is very small, but the attention it got and the fear it generated in this country have been enormous. On the one hand, then, we know the true risk of contracting Ebola, somewhere around 1 in several million. On the other hand, we *perceive* the risk as something approaching enormous. Thanks largely to the work of Daniel Kahneman and other behavioral economists, we now have a substantial amount of empirical evidence about how people form and hang on to their ideas about risk—and, for the most part, they do it very differently from how statisticians do it. A public health statistician might tell us that the risk of dying from a fall is 1 in 152 whereas the risk of dying in an airplane crash is 1 in 8,321.[21] That is a *relative risk* of 0.002, meaning that the risk of dying from a fall is 2,000 times greater than from perishing in an airplane disaster. But psychologists and behavioral economists tell us that our understanding of what these numbers mean is not straightforward. Sure, everyone can understand from this that a person is more likely to be killed slipping in the shower or falling down the stairs than flying in an airplane. But numbers like 152 and 8,321 do not have much significance for us other than to signify that one is bigger than the other.

A lot more goes into our perception of risk than the numbers that describe the actual threat. As we mentioned earlier, the human mind is naturally biased in favor of overestimating small risks and underestimating large risks. The former is the reason we buy lottery tickets and buy insurance. The latter is the reason we neglect getting a flu shot or fastening our seat belt. The decision to keep a gun in the house is another example. As Daniel Kahneman recently wrote to us, "The gun safety issue is straightforward. When you think of the safety of your home, you assume an attack. Conditional on being an attack, the gun makes you safe. No one multiplies that conditional probability by the very low probability of an attack, to compare that with the probability of an accident, which is clearly low."[22] Refusing to vaccinate a child is a classic example of this: those who fear immunization exaggerate the very, very small risk of an adverse side effect and underestimate the devastation that occurs during a measles outbreak or just how deadly whooping cough (pertussis) can be. We also get fooled by randomness—believing that something that happened by mere chance is actually a real effect.[23] Thus, if a child is vaccinated one day and gets a severe viral illness three days later we are prone to think the vaccine caused the illness, even though the two events probably happened in close proximity purely by chance. Everyone makes this mistake.

Convincing people about the relative risks of things without making them experts in biostatistics is a difficult task. And here, a little learning can be a dangerous thing. Jack recently asked a group of very educated and successful people whether the fact that there is a 1 in 1,000 chance of falling in the shower made them feel reassured or nervous. Most of them said reassured because they thought that, like a coin flip, each time they get into the shower they have the same very small risk of falling. They had absorbed the classic explanation of independent events, taught on the first day of every statistics class, represented by the odds of getting a heads or tails each time we flip a coin. But they were actually wrong. If we ask not what are the odds of tossing heads on each coin flip, which is always 1 in 2 (50%) because each toss is an independent event, but rather what are the odds of flipping at least 1 head in 100 coin flips we get a very different answer: 99%. Similarly, if the risk of falling in the shower is 1/1,000 and you take a shower every day you will probably fall at least once every 3 years. So please be careful. And clearly, trying to help people understand what is and isn't really a risk to their health requires considerable effort and novel approaches.

The last chapter in this book, "Conclusion," presents some of our recommendations for improving the recognition and use of scientific information to make health decisions. These follow naturally from our understanding of the factors that we argue contribute so much to science denial. But there is another set of overarching recommendations that we think best presented at the outset. These have to do with the need for vastly improved science education, science journalism, research into what will help nonscientists understand the nature of scientific evidence, and the recognition of all aspects of the conflict of interest conundrum. Although we will touch on these topics at many points throughout the book, we will advance our ideas on them now.

Our Desperate Need for Scientific First Responders

Analyzing the reasons for science denial in detail leads to the question of what can be done to reverse it. Clearly, new and research-proven approaches to educating the public are urgently needed if we are going to accomplish this. We have used the African Ebola epidemic (which did not, and will not, become a North American epidemic) as a recent example of public misperception about scientific evidence that ultimately proved harmful. Because of public hysteria, African Americans and Africans visiting the United States were shunned, abused, and even beaten.[24] It was initially proposed that in return for their brave service in Africa treating the victims of Ebola, healthcare workers returning home to the United States should be quarantined for a minimum of 21 days. When Dr. Craig Spencer returned to New York City after treating Ebola patients in Guinea, his fiancée and two friends with whom he had had contact were ordered into quarantine for 21 days, his apartment was sealed off, and a bowling alley he had been to in Brooklyn was shuttered. Much of this was an overreaction based on fear rather than science. Fortunately, Dr. Spencer survived.[25]

Ebola is not a public health crisis in the United States, but it does represent a public relations disaster for public health, medicine, and science. Because scientists understood that it would be highly unlikely for Ebola to get a foothold here given its mode of transmission, which makes it a not very contagious organism, they knew that the proper response was to fight the infection where it was really an epidemic, in Africa. Craig Spencer, in a very moving article he wrote after his discharge from the hospital, laments the fact that our attention was misplaced when media and politicians focused on the nonexistent threat to Americans. "Instead of being welcomed as respected humanitarians," he wrote, "my U.S. colleagues who have returned home from battling Ebola have been treated as pariahs."[26] That was wrong from two points of view. The first is, of course, a moral one—America has the most advanced medical technology in the world and we have an ethical obligation to use what we know to save the lives of people who are unable to access the benefits of modern medical science. Fulfilling this obligation is of course a complex endeavor and beyond the scope of this book, but we cannot avoid being painfully aware that Americans did not care very much about Ebola when it was limited to Liberia, Sierra Leone, Guinea, and other West African countries.

The second reason it was wrong to ignore the Ebola epidemic in Africa is more germane to our concerns here. It was always clear that a few cases of Ebola would show up in this country. Remember that we have been fed a steady diet of movies, books, and television programs in recent years in which lethal viruses suddenly emerge that kill millions of people in days and threaten to eliminate humanity. In those dramatic depictions (which usually have only a tenuous relationship to actual biology and epidemiology), a handful of very physically attractive scientists, who know better than the rest of the scientific community, courageously intervene to figure out how to stop the viral plague and save the human race. These are the kind of things that scientists tend not to read or watch or even know about, but they should because we see them all the time.

Therefore, given the fact that Ebola was going to crop up somewhere in the United States and that people are programmed to be frightened of it, the CDC should have initiated a public education campaign as soon as the African epidemic became known. Perhaps the organization did not do so because public health officials feared that bringing up the possibility that Ebola would certainly come here would frighten people and cause hysteria. If so, it was a bad decision because fear and hysteria is exactly what emerged when Thomas Duncan got sick. Hence, weeks that could have been devoted to preparing Americans to make a sensible response were wasted. Craig Spencer recognized this when he wrote, "At times of threat to our public health, we need one pragmatic response, not 50 viewpoints that shift with the proximity of the next election."[27]

An even more likely reason behind the failure of CDC and other public health and medical agencies to be proactive in dealing with America's response to Ebola is the sad fact that these groups generally do not see public education as their job. Over and over again we see the public health and scientific communities ignoring events that are guaranteed to frighten people. The scientists decide, usually correctly, that the popular explanations of such events are wrong—there is no danger—and therefore not worthy of their attention. Only after the false notions become embedded in many people's minds does the scientific community mount any meager effort to counteract it.

A good example of this occurred when Brian Hooker published an online article on August 27, 2014. In this paper, which had no coauthors, Hooker took data assembled by the CDC and previously published[28] that addressed the purported relationship between autism and vaccination and "re-analyzed" them. He used a very basic statistical test called the chi-square and concluded that African American males who had been given the MMR vaccine before age 36 months were more than 3 times more likely to have autism than African American males who received the vaccination after 36 months.

This is a shocking conclusion. Every piece of evidence previously reported failed to find any association between vaccinations and autism. Hooker claimed that "for genetic subpopulations" the MMR vaccine "may be associated with adverse events." The story went viral on the Internet and throughout social media. Almost immediately the "news" that Hooker had discovered an association between an immunization and autism in African American males led to accusations that the CDC knew about this from the beginning and deliberately chose to hide it. So-called anti-vaxxers who had been maintaining all along that vaccinations cause autism and weaken the immune system of children felt they had finally gotten the scientific confirmation for which they had been longing. Moreover, a conspiracy theory was born and the generally admired CDC plastered with scorn.

The Hooker "analysis" is actually close to nonsensical. For a variety of technical reasons having to do with study methodology and statistical inference, some of which we will mention shortly, it has absolutely no scientific validity. Indeed, the journal editors who published it retracted the article on October 3, 2014, with the following explanation:

> The Editor and Publisher regretfully retract the article as there were undeclared competing interests on the part of the author which compromised the peer review process. Furthermore, post-publication peer review raised concerns about the validity of the methods and statistical analysis, therefore the Editors no longer have confidence in the soundness of the findings. We apologize to all affected parties for the inconvenience caused.[29]

The "undisclosed" conflict of interest is the well-known fact that Hooker, the father of a child with autism, is a board member of an organization called Focus Autism, which has campaigned incessantly to assert that vaccines cause autism. Many critics rushed to point out that Hooker has spent years addressing this topic but is not himself an expert in immunology, infectious diseases, autism, or any relevant discipline. He is a chemical engineer.

Importantly, the Hooker paper was ignored by the medical, scientific, and public health communities for days. The paper itself was accessed online frequently and became the subject of reports all over the media. Journalists debated its merits and tried to get comments from scientists at the CDC. Anti-vaxxer groups went wild with self-righteous glee. Here was the smoking gun they knew all along existed. And in the midst of this was virtual silence from the experts who knew immediately the paper by Hooker was simply incorrect.

The problem is that explaining why Hooker's paper is wrong and should never have been published in the first place is a complicated task full of technical points. The original paper by DeStefano and colleagues in which these data were first reported in 2004 is not easy reading. In fact, nowhere in the paper do the exact words "We found that there is no relationship between the MMR vaccine and autism" occur.

The original investigators' hypothesis was that if MMR vaccinations caused autism, then children with autism should have received the MMR vaccine before the age when autism developed. Clearly, a vaccination given *after* a child has received a diagnosis of autism cannot be its cause. Therefore, more children with autism should have received the vaccine before age 36 months than children without autism. The results are therefore analyzed in terms of ages at which first vaccination was given, and according to figure 1 in the paper it is clear that there is no difference between the groups (see table 1). Thus the authors concluded, "In this population-based study in a large U.S. metropolitan area [Atlanta, Georgia], we found that the overall distribution of ages at first MMR vaccination among children with autism was similar to that of school-matched control children who did not have autism." In other words, there was no evidence of any relationship between MMR vaccine and autism.

TABLE 1 Comparison of Demographic Characteristics and Cognitive Levels Between Included and Excluded Autism Case Children*

Characteristic	Included Cases (N = 624)		Excluded Cases (N = 363)	
	n	%	n	%
Age group (y)				
3–5	214	34	131	36
6–10	410	66	232	64
Gender				
Male	500	80	292	80
Female	124	20	71	20
Mental retardation				
Yes	376	60	205	56
No	248	40	158	44

*Reproduced with permission from *Pediatrics*, 113, 259–266, Copyright © 2004, by the AAP.

To anyone with an advanced understanding of case-control study methods, hypothesis testing, and regression analysis, the DeStefano paper is very reassuring. To most people, however, it is probably opaque. There are multiple points at which a charlatan could seize upon the authors' honest explanations of what they did and did not do, take them out of context, and distort the meaning of the paper. Hooker went even beyond this—he took the data and did what scientists and statisticians call "data massage." If you take a big data set and query it enough times, for mathematical reasons it will sooner or later give a spurious result by chance. That is why it is improper to take a data set and chop it up into subgroups and redo the analyses. But that is essentially what Hooker did by looking separately at boys and girls and various ethnic groups. He also applied inappropriate statistical methods—simple chi-square tests are not the correct way to analyze data from a large case control study like DeStefano's.

It was not particularly difficult for us to explain these shortcomings in Hooker's analysis. We could, if asked, make them simpler or more complex. Nothing would make us happier than to have the opportunity to explain technical aspects of the DeStefano paper over and over again until nonscientists understand what is going on here. But sadly, no one from the pediatric, epidemiology, or statistics communities jumped on the opportunity the minute the Hooker paper appeared. It is uncertain how many mothers and fathers of 2- and 3-year-old children who had been on the fence about vaccinating their children decided not to do so in the days after Hooker's paper appeared online.

It has been customary for scientists, physicians, and public health experts to blame people when they follow anti-science notions. When the culprit is a charismatic leader who—with the stakes for the public so high—fails to adhere meticulously to accepted scientific norms, we agree that blame is exactly what needs to be assigned. But most people who believe science denialist ideas truly think they are protecting their and their children's health. Clearly what is desperately needed is rigorously conducted research into the best methods to educate people about scientific issues. The results may be surprising, but waiting until we are gripped with fear and swayed by incorrect ideas is obviously not an option. We need a corps of "scientific first responders" to address science denialism the minute it appears.

But Science Is Boring . . . Right?

How can we make sure everyone is equipped to make decisions based on science? It is becoming abundantly apparent which actions do *not* work to improve everyone's understanding of scientific evidence and chief among them is lecturing, haranguing, and telling people not to be so emotional. Emotion is what makes us loving, empathic human beings, capable of working together in social groups, maintaining family units and being altruistic and charitable. It is also what drives a great deal of our daily activity and powerfully influences how we make decisions. Turning it off is both unpleasant (sports fans know that in-depth analyses of every technicality during a basketball game becomes tedious and ruins the thrill of watching great athletes compete) and nearly impossible. Further, we are not interested in advocating that everyone become an automaton who obsesses over every decision and every action.

Rather, as we assert, it will be necessary to study and develop new strategies at two levels: one, to help school-age children actually like science and enjoy thinking like scientists, and two, to initiate serious research on the best way to convince adults that following scientific evidence in making choices is in their best interests. In chapter 5 on complexity we make clear that the current method of teaching science, which largely relies on forcing children to memorize facts and perform boring cookbook-style "experiments," is guaranteed to make most of them hate the subject. Furthermore, the present pedagogical approach does not give children a sense of how scientists work, what the scientific method looks like in action, or how to understand what constitutes scientific evidence. Teaching children what it means to make a scientific hypothesis, to test it, and to decide if it is correct or not, we argue, may be far more likely to both increase the number of children who actually like science and create a citizenry that can sort out scientific facts from hype.

There is already robust evidence that hands-on learning in science, in which young students do rather than simply absorb science, enhances both the enjoyment students get from science education and their proficiency with scientific concepts.[30] Two graduate students in the University of Pennsylvania chemistry department recently founded a program called Activities for Community Education in Science (ACES) in which local Philadelphia schoolchildren perform a variety of experiments in the program that are designed to be fun.[31] This approach is very different from typical lab classes that use a cookbook-style approach in which students follow a series of prescribed steps in order to get—if they do each step exactly correctly—a preordained result. A few students find the typical approach challenging, but many others get bored and frustrated. Most important, the usual lab class in high school and college science courses does not mimic the excitement of laboratory research. There is no "cookbook" for guidance when one is proceeding through a new experiment. Rather, scientists are constantly figuring out if what they are doing is leading in the right direction, if an intermediary result makes it more or less likely that the whole study will provide a meaningful result.

There are signs that some work is now being done to rectify this situation. Peter J. Alaimo and colleagues at Seattle University developed a new approach to undergraduate organic chemistry lab class in which students must "think, perform, and behave more like professional scientists."[32] In the ACES program just mentioned students and their mentors similarly focus on the concepts guiding the experiments. This restores the sense of discovery that can make otherwise tedious lab work exciting. Similar efforts are being made in colleges across the country like the Universities of California, Davis; Colorado; and North Carolina.[33] As we always stress, and as the students who designed the program well understand, we will know how successful these programs are only when they are subjected to serious evaluation research themselves.

There is even less reliable scientific information on the best way to influence adults. A large part of the problem is the persistent refusal of scientific organizations to get involved in public education. As we saw with the Ebola crisis, even otherwise impressive agencies like the CDC wait far too long to recognize when people need to be provided correct information in a formulation that can be understood and that is emotionally persuasive. We surely need public health officials who are prepared to take to the airwaves—perhaps social media—on a regular basis and who anticipate public concerns and fears. To take another example, it was recently announced that scientists determined that the radiation reaching the U.S. Pacific coast 2 years after the Japanese Fukushima meltdown is of much too low a concentration to be a health threat. It is not clear whether this information calmed the perpetrators of terrifying stories of the threat of radiation to Californians.[34] But what is needed to be sure that such frightening claims are rejected by the public are proactive campaigns carefully addressing understandable fears and explaining in clear terms that the reassuring information was gathered via extensive, exhaustive monitoring and measurement using sophisticated technology and not as part of government cover-ups.

Dan Kahan, Donald Braman, and Hank Jenkins-Smith, of Yale and Georgetown Universities and the University of Oklahoma, respectively, conducted a series of experiments that demonstrated how cultural values and predispositions influence whom we see as a scientific "expert."[35] They concluded from their work:

It is not enough to assure that scientifically sound information— including evidence of what scientists themselves believe—is widely disseminated: cultural cognition strongly motivates individuals—of all worldviews—to recognize such information as sound in a selective pattern that reinforces their cultural predispositions. To overcome this effect, communicators must attend to the cultural meaning as well as the scientific content of information.

Culture in this regard includes those that are created around an anti-science cause. People who oppose GMOs, nuclear power, or vaccinations often turn these ideas into a way of life in which a culture of opposition is created. Disrupting even one tenet of this culture is experienced by its adherents as a mortal blow to their very raison d'être.

At present, we know very little about the best ways to educate adults about science. Some of our assumptions turn out to be wrong. For example, it has long been known that the perception of risk is heightened when a warning about a potential danger is accompanied by highly emotional content. Those who oppose vaccination pepper their outcries with appeals to our most basic human sympathies by detailing cases of children who were supposedly harmed. It is a laudable human emotion that we are instantly moved by a child in distress: while other species sometimes even eat their young, humans have developed a basic instinct to do almost anything to protect or save the life of an unrelated young boy or girl. No wonder, then, that anti-vaxxer advertisements are so compelling. With this knowledge in hand, a group of scientists devised an experiment to see if confronting parents who are ambivalent about vaccination with information about the ravages of measles and other preventable infectious diseases would push them toward vaccination approval. The researchers were surprised to find that their emotionally laden messages actually made things worse: parents who were already scared of the alleged adverse side effects of immunization became more so when they were given these frightening messages.[36] We will delve a bit more into the possible reasons for this later in this book.

Similarly, inclusion of more graphic warnings about the dangers of cigarette smoking on cigarette packaging and advertisements was mandated by the Food and Drug Administration in 2012. There is some evidence that this is more effective in motivating people to stop smoking than the previous, more benign health warnings.[37] There has been a dramatic decrease in the number of Americans who smoke since the surgeon general issued the first report detailing the risks of nicotine. Nevertheless, after more than 50 years of warning the public that cigarettes kill, it is entirely unclear to what extent educational efforts contributed to that decline. All that is certain is that increasing taxes on cigarettes and enforcing rules about where smoking is allowed have been effective.[38] Scare tactics can easily backfire, as has been observed by climate scientists trying to warn us about the severe implications of global warming. Ted Nordhaus and Michael Shellenberger of the environmental research group Breakthrough Institute summarized this issue: "There is every reason to believe that efforts to raise public concern about climate change by linking it to natural disasters will backfire. More than a decade's worth of research suggests that fear-based appeals about climate change inspire denial, fatalism and polarization."[39] What is needed instead, they argue, are educational messages that stress goals that people will recognize they can actually accomplish. Scaring people may make people pray for deliverance but not take scientifically driven action.

These educational efforts must be extended to our legislators, who often claim ignorance about anything scientific. Politics frequently invades scientific decision making, and here our legislators must be far more sophisticated in understanding the difference between legitimate debates over policy and misleading ones over scientific evidence. That the earth is warming due to human-driven carbon emissions is not debatable. How to solve this problem—for example, with what combination of solar, wind, and nuclear power—is a legitimate topic of public debate. As David Shiffman once complained:

> When politicians say "I'm not a scientist," it is an exasperating evasion. . . . This response raises lots of other important questions about their decision-making processes. Do they have opinions about how best to maintain our nation's highways, bridges, and tunnels—or do they not because they're not civil engineers? Do they refuse to talk about agriculture policy on the grounds that they're not farmers?[40]

Educating politicians about science can work, as was recently shown with a project in the African country Botswana. Hoping to improve the quality of discussion, debate, and lawmaking about HIV and AIDS, members of the Botswana parliament were contacted by a research group and asked if they felt they needed more education. As reported in *Science*, the MPs "cited jargon and unexplained technical language and statistical terms as key blocks to their understanding and use of evidence."[41] They were then provided hands-on training that touched on key concepts of science like control groups, bias, and evidence. The experiment in legislator education seems to have been successful:

> The feedback from the Botswana legislators was very favorable; they asked for further session to cover the topics in more detail and for the training to be offered to other decision-makers. After the training . . . a senior parliamentarian noted that parliamentary debate—for example around the updated national HIV policy—was more sophisticated and focused on evidence.

The researchers involved in the Botswana project are quick to caution, however, that its true value will not be known until the long-term impact is formally measured. Testimonials from people involved in a project like this are a kind of one-way street. Had the legislators given an unambiguously unfavorable assessment of their experience, they would have clearly indicated that the program in its present state is unlikely to be worthwhile. A positive response, however, is less clear. It could be that the program will prove effective or that the people enrolled in it were grateful and therefore biased to give favorable responses. Even when studying science education the usual principles of the scientific method apply and uncertainty is the required initial pose.

Indeed, at present we are not certain how best to convince people that there are scientific facts involved in making health decisions and that ignoring them has terrible consequences. Hence, one of the most important things we will recommend is increased funding by the National Institutes of Health, National Science Foundation, Department of Education, CDC, FDA, and other relevant public and private agencies for science communication research. This is not the same as research on science education for youth, although that too needs a great deal more funding and attention. By science communication, we mean the ways in which scientific facts are presented so that they are convincing. Attention must also be paid to the wide variety of information sources. Traditional journalism—print, radio, and television—has sometimes fallen short in communicating science to the public. In part this is because very few journalists have more than a rudimentary understanding of scientific principles and methods. One study showed that much of the information offered in medical talk shows has no basis in fact.[42] But perhaps a bigger problem rests with the perception that people are interested only in controversies. Journalists might try to excuse the dissemination of sensationalistic versions of science by insisting that they are providing only what people want to hear. After all, no one is forcing the public to pay for and read their publications. But the result of this kind of reporting is the fabrication of scientific controversies when in fact none exist. Journalists must learn that the notion of "fair balance" in science does not mean that outliers should get the same level of attention as mainstream scientists. These outliers are not lonely outcasts crying out the truth from the desert but rather simply wrong. Science and politics are not the same in this regard.

Another mistake found in some science journalism is accepting the absence of evidence as signifying the evidence of absence. Let us say for example that a study is published in which a much touted, promising new treatment for cancer is found to work no better than an already available medication. The conclusion of the scientific article is "We failed to find evidence that 'new drug' is better than 'old drug.'" The headline of the article in the newspaper, however, is "New Drug Does Not Work for Cancer." Demonstrating that one drug is better than another involves showing that the rate of response to the first drug is not only larger than to the second drug but that it is *statistically significantly* larger. Let's say for example that 20 patients with cancer are randomized so that 10 get the new drug and 10 get the old drug. The people who get the new drug survive 9 months after starting treatment and the people who get the old drug survive for only 3 months. That difference of 6 months may seem important to us, but because there are so few people in the trial and given the technical details of statistical analysis it is quite likely that the difference won't be statistically significant. Hence, the researchers are obligated to say they can't detect a difference. But in the next sentence of their conclusion they will certainly state that "a future study with a larger number of patients may well show that 'new drug' offers a survival advantage."

In this case, however, the journalist, unlike the scientist, cannot accept uncertainty about whether the drug does or doesn't work. A story must be written with a firm conclusion. Hence, the incorrect conclusion that the drug doesn't work, period. When further research later on finds that the drug does work to significantly improve survival, perhaps for a subgroup of people with upper respiratory cancer, the journalist has moved on to a different story and the news does not see the light of day. Journalists need education in the proper communication of science and the scientific method.

Today, of course, we get most of our information from all kinds of sources. Here again, public education is vitally needed. The idea that the first result that pops up in a Google search is necessarily the best information must be systematically eradicated from people's minds. The Internet is a fabulous development that facilitates, among other things, writing books like this one. But it is also loaded with polemical content, misinformation, and distortions of the truth when it comes to science. Gregory Poland and Robert Jacobson at the Mayo Clinic did a simple search 15 years ago and found 300 anti-vaccine Internet sites.[43] Helping people avoid merely getting confirmation for their incorrect beliefs must be the topic of extensive research.

The Conflict of Interest Conflict

Whom we ultimately select to carry out this education will also be tricky. The charismatic leaders of science denialist groups often have impressive scientific credentials, although they are usually not in the field most relevant to the area of science under discussion. Still, simply having an MD, MPH, or PhD in a scientific field is not sufficient to distinguish a science denialist from a scientist. It is clear that the people who carry out this education should themselves be charismatic in the sense that they can speak authoritatively and with emotion, that they truly care about educating the public, and that they are not angry at "ignorance," arrogant, or condescending.

One of the most controversial areas, of course, will be "purity," by which we mean a near complete absence of potential conflicts of interest. A very prominent rallying cry by science denialists is the charge that our health and well-being is threatened by corporations and their paid lackeys. Whoever disagrees with a science denialist is frequently accused of being "bought and paid for" by a drug company, an energy company, a company that makes genetically modified seeds, and so forth.

There is no question that money is a powerful motivator to ignore bias in scientific assessments. Although pharmaceutical companies insist otherwise, it is clear that their promotional and marketing activity directed at doctors influences prescribing behavior.[44] Doctors and scientists on expert panels that design professional guidelines for treatment of many medical disorders often receive funding for their research or for service on advisory boards from drug companies that make the same drugs that are recommended for use in those guidelines. Studies of medications that are funded by pharmaceutical companies are more likely to show positive results than are those funded by nonprofit sources like the NIH. As someone who once accepted considerable amounts of money from pharmaceutical companies for serving on advisory boards and giving lectures, Jack can attest to the sometimes subtle but unmistakable impact such funding has on a doctor's or scientist's perspective. It is not a matter of consciously distorting the truth, but rather being less likely to see the flaw in a drug made by a company that is providing funding.[45]

Scientific journals now require extensive disclosure of any such relationships before accepting a paper. Sunshine laws are currently being passed that require drug companies to make known all the physicians to whom they give money. Other scientists and healthcare professionals are rightly suspicious of studies funded by pharmaceutical companies; studies that result in a negative outcome for the company's product are generally not published, and sometimes negative aspects of a drug are obscured in what otherwise seems a positive report.

The issue is not, of course, restricted to scientists and doctors. A recent article in the *Harvard Business Review* noted that "Luigi Zingales, a professor at Chicago's Booth School of Business, found that economists who work at business schools or serve on corporate boards are more supportive of high levels of executive pay than their colleagues."[46] An important aspect to this finding is that the economists, just like doctors in a similar position, truly believed that they were immune to such influence. People who take money from corporations have the same "I am in control" bias that we see when they insist they are safer driving a car than flying in a plane because they are in control of only the former: "Money may influence other people's opinions, but I am fully in control of this and completely objective."

Corporate support for science is always going to run the risk of at least creating the impression of bias if not actually causing it outright. Elizabeth Whelan, who founded the American Council on Science and Health, was an important figure in demanding that public policy involving health be based only on sound science. She decried regulations that lacked firm scientific support and correctly challenged the notion that a substance that causes an occasional cancer in a cancer-prone rat should automatically be labeled a human toxin. She famously decried the banning of foods "at the drop of a rat." Yet despite all of the important advocacy she did on behalf of science in the public square, her work was always criticized because it received major corporate financing. As noted in her *New York Times* obituary, "Critics say that corporations have donated precisely because the [American Council on Science and Health's] reports often support industry positions."[47] The fact that Whelan and her council accepted corporate money does not, of course, automatically invalidate their opinions; and even when they made a wrong call, as they did in supporting artificial sweeteners,[48] it is not necessarily because manufacturers of artificial sweeteners paid for that support. Corporate support, however, will forever cast a shadow over Whelan's scientific legacy.

The problem of obscure financial incentives also infects the antiscience side, although this is rarely acknowledged. Figure 1 is used by a group called Credo Action as part of their campaign against GMOs. It describes itself as "a social change organization that supports activism and funds progressive nonprofits—efforts made possible by the revenues from our mobile phone company, CREDO Mobile." But what is Credo Mobile? It is a wireless phone company that markets cell phones and wireless phone plans, offers a credit card, and asks potential customers to choose them over "big telecom companies." In other words, it uses social action to advertise its products. Customers might think it is a nonprofit organization, but it is not. We agree with some of the positions Credo takes and disagree with others, but that is beside the point. In their anti-GMO work, they are a for-profit cell phone company opposing a for-profit agriculture company. It takes a fair amount of digging to find that out.

So far, we have focused on conflicts of interests that involve money, but there are a number of problems with the exclusive focus on financial conflicts of interest. First of all, just because a corporation paid for

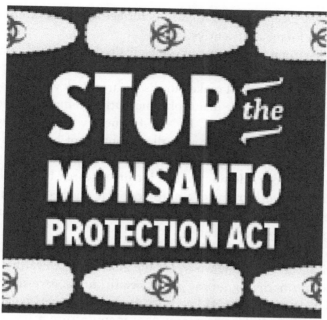

FIGURE 1 Advertisement from Credo Mobile, a for-profit company that uses social action to promote its products.

Source: From http://act.credoaction.com/sign/monsanto_protection_act

a study or makes a product does not automatically deem it a tainted study or dangerous product. Most of the medications we take are in fact safe and effective. Cases of acute food toxicity are fortunately infrequent. Some pesticides and herbicides are not harmful to humans, only to insects, rodents, and invasive weeds. The involvement of corporate money rightly makes us suspicious and insistent on safeguards to ensure that finances have not led to shortcuts or unethical behavior, but it does not justify a reflexive conclusion that corruption is involved.

Another problem is that focusing only on financial conflicts of interests ignores the many other factors that can cause bias in science. In the Brian Hooker example we discussed earlier in this chapter the bias was in the form of belonging to an organization with an agenda that does not permit dissent. Hooker's views are suspect not because he is getting money from a large corporation but because he belongs to what appears to be a cult of believers who steadfastly refuse to acknowledge anything that contradicts their views. Deep emotional reasons for being biased can be just as strong as a financial incentive.

We are strong proponents of complete disclosure of *all* competing interests.

In that spirit, we will make our disclosures. Jack worked as a consultant to almost all the major pharmaceutical companies and some minor ones for many years. He was frequently paid by drug companies to give lectures, and a small percentage of his research was also funded by drug companies. He stopped taking money from drug companies in 2003. He was funded for his research by the National Institutes of Health from 1982 until 2006. He has been an employee of private medical schools, a private healthcare company, and of the New York State government.

Sara is an employee of a large, multinational healthcare and pharmaceutical company. She works for the global public health division, involved in improving global public health in resource-limited settings. The vast majority of her work does not involve pharmaceutical products at all. Her company does manufacture a few vaccines and antibiotics, but this is a relatively small part of their business in which Sara does not work. She developed her views on the safety of vaccinations before joining the company.

We are also clear about our positions on the topics we cover. We think every child should receive all of the vaccinations recommended by the American Academy of Pediatrics, that no one should have a gun in his or her home, that antibiotics are overprescribed, that nuclear energy and genetically modified foods are safe and necessary when the appropriate safeguards are in place and carefully maintained, that ECT is a safe and effective treatment for severe depression, and that unpasteurized milk should be outlawed. We hope our readers do not hold these opinions against us. Our opinions are based on our reading of the scientific literature. Many of them are unpopular among our closest friends and family. We also hope our readers will always bear in mind that the main focus of this book is not to argue back and forth about vaccinations, GMOs, or nuclear power but rather to present a framework to understand why people deny scientific evidence and how this situation can be improved.

We believe that without the capacity to make decisions based on science, we are doomed to waste time and precious resources and to place ourselves and our children at great risk. This is why we believe the time has come to more fully explore the intricacies of irrational health beliefs and the responses the medical and health communities have employed. This is why we have undertaken to write this book. Elucidating causes of irrational health decisions and what to do about them is not easy, and we certainly do not claim to have all the answers. But it is essential that we try, since we can say, without exaggeration, that these decisions frequently mean the difference between life and death.

Just a word on the title: *Denying to the Grave* signifies two themes that are central to this book. The first highlights the potential consequences of denying what science tells us. If we refuse to vaccinate our children, some of them will become very sick with otherwise preventable illnesses. If we take antibiotics unnecessarily, we will promote the spread of resistant bacterial strains capable of causing severe disease and even death. In each case, refusing to accept sound scientific evidence can produce dire outcomes. But we want to make clear once more that this first point, as important as it is to our work, is not where we spend most of our time. The data are overwhelming for each of the scientific issues we use as examples in *Denying to the Grave*, and extensive reviews of the evidence are not our central purpose. Rather, it is on the second meaning of *Denying to the Grave* that we focus most of our attention: the willingness of people to "take to the grave" their scientific misconceptions in the face of abundant evidence that they are wrong and placing themselves in danger doing so. We are less concerned with convincing our readers that they should vaccinate their children (of course they should) than with trying to understand why some intelligent, well-meaning people hold tenaciously to the notion that vaccines are dangerous. The same principle holds for GMOs, nuclear power, antibiotics, pasteurization, electroconvulsive therapy, and all the other examples we call upon to illustrate this puzzling phenomenon.

We do not claim to be complete experts on all of the topics discussed in the book, but we are expert at discerning the difference between good and bad evidence. This is a skill we hope many of our readers will strive to attain. And of course, we do not claim to be immune from the psychological tricks that can sometimes cause any one of us to disbelieve evidence. No one is. We simply humbly offer what we do know to improve the way we all think about denial of evidence. As such, this book is aimed at a variety of audiences, from public health and medical professionals to science journalists to scientists to politicians and policymakers. Most important, we hope this book will be of use to everyone who is or has ever been confused about scientific debates they have read about in the news or heard about from friends. We count ourselves in this group, as well as many of our close friends and family, and we hope you will join us in this journey to try to understand where this confusion comes from and what to do about it.

Conspiracy Theories

C ONSPIRACIES ARE MYSTERIOUS. WE THINK IT IS REASONABLE TO say, even without any data to support it, that most people have never been part of a conspiracy or even known a person who has. It seems that in ordinary life getting even a moderately sized group of people who all agree on something together, finding time to meet, and then planning and actually implementing a secret operation over a long period of time would be fairly difficult. Getting a few people together to plan a surprise birthday party and keeping the plans secret until the actual event is difficult enough. Many of us believed at one point or another as we were growing up that our parents were conspiring against us, but today's parents rarely have the time or energy for even that much underhanded activity.

Nevertheless, we are routinely asked to believe that large, well-organized, and focused conspiracies exist that, in order to maximize their profits and scope of influence, have as their goal the destruction of our health and well-being. Every charismatic leader we will describe in the next chapter claims to be the victim of at least one such conspiracy. In the health and medical fields, the alleged conspirators usually include some combination of organized medicine, mainstream academic science and public health, the government, and large pharmaceutical and other companies. Even Wayne LaPierre, the leader of the National Rifle Association with its vast economic resources and ties to the gun manufacturing industry, portrays himself as the victim of a conspiracy of left-wing politicians, the media, and the federal government, all of whom, he would have us believe, are intent on denying Americans their Second Amendment rights, thereby exposing us innocent citizens to bands of marauding, well-armed criminals.[1] According to the leaders of conspiracy theory groups, "Most conspiracies are . . . invisible to the vast majority of sheeplike citizens who go grazing through the pasture of life, never suspecting the evil wolves lurking behind the rocks of everyday occurrences"[2] Therefore, the conspiracy theory leaders tell us, they themselves are indispensable for our very survival. Although we frequently criticize the scientific community in this book for treating us as if we were ubiquitously stupid, it is often these conspiracy group leaders who act as if we are all fools.

You may detect from the tone we have taken in introducing this subject of conspiracy theories that we find them to be largely misguided at best and dangerous at worst. Indeed, as we review the supposed conspiracies that science deniers invoke to warn us against vaccinating our children, eating GMO-based foods, undergoing ECT if we are severely depressed, or shunning nuclear power, it will become clear that in these cases no such conspiracies actually exist. Hence, it would be so simple if we could conclude that one way to be sure science deniers are wrong is to note whether they are invoking secret and well-organized conspiracies as their enemies; if they are, we may dismiss them.

Maybe It's a Conspiracy After All

In reality, we cannot accept the foregoing conclusion in any sense as a general rule because some conspiracies do in fact exist and some of them have indeed been harmful to human health. Perhaps the most egregious example of a real conspiracy in recent times was the collaboration of tobacco companies and a handful of scientists to deny the fact that cigarette smoking causes cancer and many other serious diseases. Let us imagine that in 1965 a crusader goes on the radio and television talk show circuit insisting that nicotine is a powerfully addicting substance and that smoking cigarettes is a deadly addiction. Furthermore, this crusader declares that tobacco companies, which usually compete against each other, had joined forces to finance a cadre of scientists with impressive credentials to promote false and misleading science supposedly showing that cigarettes are harmless. In addition, this conspiracy of tobacco companies and scientists was prepared to use its vast financial resources and scientific influence to ruin the scientific careers of anyone who dared claim otherwise and even to spread around lavish political contributions (not much different in this case from bribes) to government officials in order to induce them to back away from legislating against tobacco products.

Before we comment on the legitimacy of our imaginary anti-tobacco crusader's claims, let's quickly mention another conspiracy theory. A gastroenterologist named Dr. Andrew Wakefield claims that childhood vaccines are dangerous, capable of causing autism and other developmental abnormalities. Dr. Wakefield insists that pharmaceutical companies who make vaccines and usually compete against each other have joined forces to finance a cadre of scientists and pediatricians with impressive credentials to promote false and misleading science showing that vaccines are safe. Furthermore, this conspiracy of pharmaceutical companies and scientists is prepared to use its vast financial resources and scientific influence to ruin anyone who dares to claim otherwise and to bribe government officials and medical societies with contributions in order to get them to support widespread vaccination programs.

There is no question that in the first example (Big Tobacco) the imaginary crusader would have been absolutely correct and in the second Dr. Wakefield is absolutely wrong. The horrible saga of the tobacco industry and its scientific cronies shamelessly obscuring the clear evidence that cigarettes are addictive and lethal is one of the greatest blots on industrial and scientific conduct in our history. No one knows how many millions of people who died from the effects of smoking cigarettes might have been saved if that conspiracy had not delayed the public's finally understanding the truth about nicotine and government's passing stiff tax laws that discourage the purchase of cigarettes. On the other hand, Dr. Wakefield's conspiracy is a fantasy. The scientific evidence that vaccines are safe and effective is overwhelming and there has never been any need for pharmaceutical companies to engage in secret activities to promote them. Doctors know that vaccination is

an evidence-based practice, and lots of people who have no financial stake in the vaccine industry—like the entire world of public
health officials—highly recommend vaccination. In short, people
die from smoking cigarettes and lives are saved by vaccination.

But looking again at these two scenarios, we notice that the descriptions of them sound awfully similar. Back in January 1964 when
Dr. Luther Terry issued the first Surgeon General's report about
smoking, about half of all American men and one-third of women
were smokers. They did not just read the report, agree that the evidence it synthesized was solid, and quit smoking. In fact, it took
years before smoking rates actually began to decline, during which
time the tobacco industry did everything it could to counteract the
message with a ruthless disinformation campaign.[3] It took some very
dedicated crusaders who were brave enough to face down the oppro-
brium of the tobacco industry and its hired hand scientists before an
American public that had associated smoking with "Joe Camel," the
"Marlboro Man," and "You've Come a Long Way, Baby" realized
that they were being victimized by a conspiracy that was perfectly
happy to see it be exterminated as long as profits remained high.
Naomi Oreskes and Erik M. Conway lay out for us in gory detail the
shocking collaboration of some highly respected scientists with the
tobacco industry as they attempted to convince us that there is no
link between cigarette smoking and cancer:

> Millions of pages of documents released during tobacco litigation
> demonstrate these links. They show the crucial role that scientists
> played in sowing doubt about the links between smoking and health
> risks. These documents—which have scarcely been studied except by
> lawyers and a handful of academics—also show that the same strat-
> egy was applied not only to global warming, but to a laundry list of
> environmental and health concerns, including asbestos, secondhand
> smoke, acid rain, and the ozone layer.[4]

Chris Mooney and Sheril Kirshenbaum trace the origins of suspi-
ciousness about large corporations to the early 1970s.

> Not only did the new mood of "questioning authority" include the
> questioning of science, but there was often good reason for skepti-
> cism. The environmental and consumer movements, spearheaded
> by the likes of Rachel Carson and Ralph Nader, brought home the

realization that science wasn't always beneficial. Seemingly wonderful technologies—DDT, chlorofluorocarbons—could have nasty, unforeseen consequences. A narrative began to emerge about "corporate science": driven by greed, conducted without adequate safeguards, placing profits over people.[5]

In that light, then, how do we know that Dr. Terry was right but Dr. Wakefield is wrong? More important for our purposes here, how does a nonscientist consumer figure out that one person with "Dr." in front of his or her name is to be believed while another misleads us with false findings? Some conspiracies are real phenomena, while others are the concoctions of manipulative charismatic leaders who use them as a tool to advance their dangerous agendas. We acknowledge from the outset of this discussion that we will not be able to provide easy guideposts by which to make these distinctions. And these distinctions are often easily made only in retrospect, after all the facts are in. Consider the following:

- A conspiracy was behind the assassination of President Lincoln but not President Kennedy.
- A conspiracy is maintained to perpetuate the belief that high-fat diets are directly related to cardiovascular disease but is not behind the scientific consensus that foods that contain GMOs are perfectly safe.
- Conspirators hid the fact that General Motors cars had faulty ignition systems leading to several deaths, but there is no conspiracy among psychiatrists—or electric power companies—to promote ECT as a treatment for severe depression.
- A conspiracy is behind the attempt to subvert scientific evidence that conclusively demonstrates global warming to be a real and present danger, but the relative safety of nuclear energy does not need conspirators to give us honest guidance.
- A conspiracy was engineered in the Watergate scandal in an attempt to discredit the Democratic Party, but there is no conspiracy behind the scientific work proving that gun ownership is dangerous.

These five examples fall into different fields—history, nutrition science, product safety, energy science, and politics. The intriguing thing is that when we list them the way we have, there is really no obvious rule to determine which one in each pair is true and which is not. If conspirators plotted to kill one president, why couldn't there be a conspiracy behind the assassination of another one? If doctors and scientists could be so wrong about eating milk, butter, and eggs, couldn't they be equally wrong about genetically modified corn, wheat, and rice? If a company deliberately hid the dangers lurking in the use of one of its products, couldn't another group do exactly the same thing? If all this business about climate change, fossil fuels, and destroying the ozone layer is really smoke and mirrors created by some scientists to keep their grant funding rolling in, as the conspiracy theorists assert,[6] then perhaps those who tell us that nuclear power plants really don't represent a danger are also just trying to maximize their incomes. And if even the president of the United States could get himself involved in a conspiracy, then how do we know that politicians who promote gun control, like Michael Bloomberg and Gabby Giffords, don't also have some underhanded plot up their sleeves? This chapter attempts to answer some of these questions and explores why we are so prone to believing that the world is conspiring against us.

The Victim Mentality

It may help to understand something about why we are prone to gravitate toward conspiracy theories, even though most of us have never been in one and therefore have no firsthand knowledge of how they form or function. Only recently have social scientists and psychologists begun to perform experiments trying to understand what is behind conspiracy theories, and some of the information these preliminary studies have yielded is fascinating.

One of the striking characteristics of the charismatic leaders described in the next chapter is their penchant for describing themselves as victims of conspiracies. These anti-science leaders want to be seen as courageous lone wolves who are crying out against powerful and malevolent forces. They also represent themselves as belonging to a higher moral order than their opponents, who generally are depicted as ruthless and money-craving. Their messages about conspiracies can be terrifying and infuriating. In this "us" versus "them" contest, the conspiracy theorist tries to make us believe that if we don't follow his/her lead, our very survival will be threatened. In writing about HIV denialism, Seth Kalichman nicely describes the process by which the culture of scientific denialism and victimhood, whether genuinely felt or feigned, leads to conspiracism:

> A feature of denialism, at least at its root, is the tendency to think of the denialist position as beleaguered, and under attack and in a minority that has to stave off the assaults of the vast wrong-thinking majority. As a consequence, those involved in denialism often, in the other justifications for their position, declare their strong allegiance to the principle of free speech. Interestingly, then, denialists often set themselves up as plucky underdogs, battling for their rights to speak the truth against a tide of misinformation and, as often as not, conspiracies aimed at keeping them silent.[7]

How interesting it is to find out, then, that people who believe in conspiracies do so because they believe that they themselves would conspire if given the opportunity. Karen M. Douglas and Robbie M. Sutton of the School of Psychology at the University of Kent reported on some of their experiments in a paper titled "Does It Take One to Know One? Endorsement of Conspiracy Theories Is Influenced by Personal Willingness to Conspire." Based on previous research, Douglas and Sutton wondered if "those who have relatively few moral scruples about conspiring may be less likely to think that others would be deterred from conspiring, at least on moral grounds" and therefore set out to measure research participants' level of "Machiavellianism," a trait associated with "willingness to exploit others for personal gain." Jack has often said that in psychology and psychiatry "there is a scale to measure anything and everything," and indeed it turns out that there is a validated scale to measure one's level of Machiavellianism, called the MACH-IV scale. Douglas and Sutton found that the more Machiavellian a person is, the more willing he or she is to believe in conspiracy theories. Douglas and Sutton concluded, "These studies suggest that people who have more lax personal morality may endorse conspiracy theories to a greater extent because they are, on average, more willing to participate in the conspiracies themselves." [8] Thus, far from existing on a higher moral plane, conspiracy theorists on average seem to be people who "project" onto others their own openness toward conspiring. This dynamic, which anti-science conspiracy theorists would of course surely deny, may be manifest in the tendency of many charismatic leaders to form organizations with fancy-sounding names to support their causes.

This, then, may be one clue to picking out the phony conspiracy theories. Do they involve a charismatic leader who is him- or herself prone to setting up organizations that are tightly controlled by the leader, deliberate in secret, bully their opponents, and distort scientific findings? Does it seem as if the one who is promulgating a conspiracy theory is him- or herself prone to conspiring? We are reminded of Douglas and Sutton's comment that "those who have relatively few moral scruples about conspiring may be less likely to think that others would be deterred from conspiring, at least on moral grounds."

Still, most of us are prone to more subtle forms of conspiracy theories, as when we believe that the CDC is just not telling the truth about how Ebola is transmitted. So what drives a regular person to latch onto conspiracy-like beliefs?

A Dangerous Sense of Powerlessness

An important motivation fueling affiliation with conspiracy theories is the drive to overcome the feeling of powerlessness. After all, conspiracy theories assign blame to secret, powerful, and malevolent forces for things we feel we cannot control and therefore both give us an explanation for what is going on and somewhat ironically let us off the hook for doing anything about it. If the conspiracy involves the government, big corporations, and the entire healthcare profession, then no individual need feel remiss if he or she is not doing anything about the perceived problem. This makes the entry of a charismatic leader who claims to have the ability to fight back against the conspiracy an attractive option.

Studies have shown that people who feel that they lack control over situations are prone to *illusory pattern perception*, essentially seeing what is not really there. In a series of six experiments, Jennifer A. Whitson at the University of Texas, Austin, and Adam D. Galinsky, now at Columbia University, showed that study participants who lacked control over a situation saw interrelationships in random stimuli, thus creating illusory patterns out of deliberately meaningless information.[9] Among these illusory patterns were conspiracy theories. Whitson and Galinsky also showed that when the participants were given an opportunity to express self-affirmation—that is, to review their own beliefs and values—the tendency to draw these false correlations was substantially reduced. They conclude, "When individuals were made to feel psychologically secure after lacking control, they were less prone to the perception of illusory patterns." Exposure to information that supports a conspiracy theory has been shown to reduce motivation to participate in political activities, and this effect was mainly due in one experiment to feelings of powerlessness created by the information.[10]

Nor are we particularly selective about which conspiracy theories we subscribe to. Viren Swami, who works at both the University of Westminster in London and HELP University College in Kuala Lumpur, Malaysia, and his colleagues studied agreement with conspiracy theories concerning the July 7, 2005, bombings in the London public transportation system and found that "the strongest predictor of belief in 7/7 conspiracy theories was belief in other general conspiracy theories."[11] Other characteristics of willingness to agree with conspiracy theories in this study included higher political cynicism, greater support for democratic principles, more negative attitude to authority, and lower self-esteem.

Fear Jumps in Where Mistrust Already Exists

A key element in people's willingness to accept a conspiracy theory in making a healthcare decision is general mistrust and disillusionment with science.[12] Belief in conspiracy theories also tends to coincide with mistrust of science.[13] These findings have somewhat dire implications for the usual ways we try to counteract the conspiracy theorists. As researchers Jolley and Douglas note,

> Because beliefs in conspiracy theories in general are associated with a mistrust of scientific claims, interventions that cite claims by scientists and medical professionals may also meet with suspicion. Such attempts at intervention may therefore fail on people who are sympathetic to a variety of conspiracy claims.[14]

Hence, merely telling people the facts can actually serve to exacerbate the problem. For example, if one believes (a) that psychiatric drugs and ECT are universally harmful and (b) that a conspiracy of drug companies, the government, and organized psychiatry is deliberately covering up that fact in order to make money, then getting psychiatrists—no matter how prestigious they may be—to explain the true state of affairs to the public feeds directly into the conspiracists' hands. "Here again," they will tell us, "is a psychiatrist who has a vested financial interest in prescribing medications telling you they are safe. Don't even listen to him or her."

Most psychiatrists who received drug company honoraria to speak to other doctors about the benefits of new psychiatric medication give their reasons as something like this: the drugs have been shown in scientifically rigorous studies to be effective and to have acceptable levels of adverse side effects; they have been approved by the U.S. Food and Drug Administration after careful review; so why not get paid to talk about them?[15] The fact that doctors take money from drug companies to talk about the virtues of those companies' brand-name drugs does not, of course, mean the drugs are *prima facie* dangerous or that there is any conspiracy afoot. But even the *appearance* of such a conflict of interest is disillusioning to us. To make things worse, it turns out that although psychiatric drugs are indeed helpful for many patients with moderate to severe levels of illness, their effectiveness has sometimes been exaggerated and their risks downplayed by some of the pharmaceutical companies that produce them.

The cautionary note here is obvious: opponents of healthcare conspiracy theories are so automatically suspect that they must be beyond reproach and totally free of any hint of conflict of interest; they must be "squeaky clean." This is vitally important because a lot is at stake in combatting conspiracy theories in healthcare. Conspiracy theories unfortunately play a significant role in dissuading people from making lifesaving choices. Laura Bogart of Harvard University and her colleagues showed that belief in conspiracy theories was a significant reason that African American men with HIV infection did not take antiretroviral medications that had been prescribed for them.[16] In this vicious cycle, then, conspiracy theorists impugn the honesty of scientists, such as those who have proven beyond any doubt that antiretroviral medications are effective and necessary treatments for people infected with HIV. The scientists then fight back, only to face the charge that they are acting true to form, supporting ideas they are paid to support and not necessarily those that are scientifically sound. A very profitable industry selling worthless home remedies for HIV infection grew up around HIV denialism, but a fact like that is often raised mainly by scientists and doctors who themselves take money from large, established corporations like drug companies. Despite the fact that in a case like antiretroviral medications for HIV there are clear right and wrong sides, media too often present the situation as if scientists were conducting a legitimate scientific debate. Peter Duesberg, an avid HIV denialist, is given equal weight with a scientist who argues that HIV is the cause of AIDS and that antiretroviral drugs are the medically proven treatment. Duesberg can charge that his opponents receive funding from drug companies that make antiretroviral drugs and therefore nothing that they say has any merit. The men in Laura Bogart's study reading these things are bound to wonder who is correct, and those already prone to believing conspiracy theories and mistrusting science will teeter toward the dangerous decision to stop taking their medications.

Preying on the Most Vulnerable

It has sometimes been argued that belief in conspiracy theories is a logical response to complex issues that a nonspecialist cannot easily understand. The conspiracy theory supplies a readily grasped explanation that has the additional powers of emotional urgency and aligning the recipient with a cause. It is important to note, however, that society's most vulnerable people are most likely to be swayed by such theories. Marina Abalakina-Paap was at New Mexico State University when she and her colleagues published a study showing "no support for the idea that people believe in conspiracies because they provide simplified explanations of complex events."[17] A tendency to "paranoid ideation" may also be a factor,[18] although it is incorrect and counterproductive to label people who believe conspiracy theories as ubiquitously psychotic and responding to paranoid delusions. Rather, as has been shown on many occasions, people who feel powerless and have low self-esteem and low levels of trust are the easiest prey of conspiracy theorists. These are important considerations to bear in mind when devising strategies to counteract conspiracy theories. A person with low self-esteem will be resistant to overly technical scientific arguments that have the not-so-hidden message "We are scientists and you are not, so even though you are not smart enough to understand what we are telling you, believe us anyway."

The issue is not merely providing an explanation that people understand but rather an explanation that makes them feel in control. As Ted Goertzel of Rutgers University notes in his excellent article "Conspiracy Theories in Science," "A conspiracy theory gives believers someone tangible to blame for their perceived predicament, instead of blaming it on impersonal or abstract social forces."[19] For many years, parents of children with cerebral palsy were told that the cause of this tragic disorder involving the central nervous system was a lack of oxygen during labor and delivery. Obstetricians were held accountable by tort lawyers, who often won huge malpractice awards for their clients. It is clearly heartbreaking and burdensome to have a child with cerebral palsy, and blaming the doctor who delivered the child no doubt offered some solace to the parents. Moreover, it seemed like an easy explanation—the vulnerable newborn's brain receives too little oxygen during the delivery, resulting in damage to delicate nerve cells and permanent neurological and developmental abnormalities. It turns out, however, that in most cases events that occur during delivery are not the cause of cerebral palsy. What causes it? The answer is the same as it is for so many disorders involving the brain: no one knows for sure, but it appears to be a host of factors, some of which are genetic. As we will discuss in chapter 4, these kinds of unknowns are naturally difficult for people to accept and we tend to want to find a cause in which we can believe instead. All of those obstetricians who lost multimillion dollar malpractice cases when juries were bombarded with emotion-ridden displays of disabled children were generally being blamed for something totally out of their control. But it is so much easier to stick blame for a tragic outcome on a single person than to grapple with the uncertainties of "many different factors" as the cause. Again, it is not simply that parents were unable to understand the more complicated, albeit accurate explanation, but rather that assigning blame to a person gives them a sense of control over the situation. They now have something to do—be angry at the doctor and perhaps sue him or her. This gets at the emotional features of believing in conspiracy theories and indicates why simply throwing more information at people does not work.

Manipulating Our Emotions

In conspiracy theory formation, we also see at play what Daniel Kahneman, Paul Slovic, and others have called the *affect heuristic*. Our minds are programmed to respond more strongly to emotional appeals and vivid presentations than to dry facts and statistical analyses. If we are asked how we feel about nuclear power, we easily summon up images of atomic bomb clouds and nuclear power plant meltdowns. The technology strikes us as scary. More difficult would be to review the data on the actual risks posed by different forms of energy production. To do so yields a surprising result: because it contributes to outdoor air pollution, energy derived from coal and oil produces more disease and death than does energy derived from nuclear power.[20] In fact, energy produced by burning coal is responsible for 15 times as many accidental deaths as nuclear energy. According to the World Health Organization (WHO), air pollution now accounts for one of every eight deaths in the world, an estimated 7 million deaths in 2012.[21] And of course, burning fossil fuels contributes to global warming whereas nuclear energy does not. But it takes some digging to get these facts and quite a bit of thought. We have to understand that burning fossil fuels releases pollutants in the air, which increases the risk and severity of respiratory diseases like asthma. Then we have to understand that asthma can be a deadly illness. At the same time, we have to be able to examine the data showing that catastrophic nuclear power plant accidents are rare events and that those that have occurred actually resulted in fewer health problems or deaths than expected. This does not mean, of course, that nuclear power is a panacea. The issue of where and how to store nuclear waste for power plants is a plaguing one, and there are other safety and security risks that need attention. Most important, the cost of building new nuclear reactors is prohibitive, so steps must be taken to make them economically viable. Solving these issues can be done, but it will require very careful scientific and environmental science, political will, and public understanding. It is much easier to ignore the risks of burning coal, oil, and natural gas and to shut down nuclear power plants than to have to think about all of these numbers and equations.

When we face a hard question for which only slow, time-consuming deliberation will yield an answer we are prone to fall back on emotional judgments; in other words, we employ the affect heuristic. "The affect heuristic simplifies our lives by creating a world that is much tidier than reality," Kahneman writes. "Good technologies have few costs in the imaginary world we inhabit, bad technologies have no benefits, and all decisions are easy. In the real world, of course, we often face painful tradeoffs between benefits and costs."[22] As we discuss at other points in this book, simple, vivid, emotional messages, especially when they evoke unpleasant feelings like fear and disgust, activate more primitive regions of the human brain and inhibit the more rational, contemplative regions. It makes sense that these primitive regions, which include structures such as the nucleus accumbens, amygdala, and insula, are more rapidly and easily engaged. They evolved to make us take action under circumstances of life-threatening danger. If smoke is filling the room you are in, it is not important for you to figure out where it is coming from, whether the amount of smoke and its rate of filling the room are likely to pose a threat, and the biology by which smoke inhalation causes asphyxiation; instead, you had better quickly exit that room! We react to nuclear power as if it is smoke filling the room: we see the technology as potentially life-threatening and our response is "Shut it down."

It's All in Your Head

Under ordinary circumstances the more evolved part of the human brain, the prefrontal cortex (PFC), can be recruited to exert reason over emotion, albeit with some effort. Antonio Damascio, who has done groundbreaking research in understanding the impact of brain function on emotion and behavior, observed that people with damage to the ventromedial portion of the PFC—an area that is located in the front of the brain, toward the bottom, and in the middle—results in an inability to attach feelings and emotions with actual consequences.[23] But very strong emotional reactions, like extreme fear, also serve to inhibit this part of the brain. The result is an inability to control emotional impulses. Anti-science conspiracy theories are characterized by a great deal of dramatic, emotional content. Everything is couched in terms of inflammatory words and phrases—brain damage, armed intruders, radiation sickness, rich corporate giants, and so forth.

If we think of conspiracy theorists' ability to convince us what to think as a kind of social influence, we can understand the phenomenon in terms of recent brain research. For example, Micah G. Edelson of the Department of Neurobiology at the Weizmann Institute of Science in Israel and colleagues from England and New York published the results of an experiment in which participants watched a movie and then answered questions about it.[24] Next, brain imaging was conducted while the participants were again asked the questions but this time after receiving false answers to the questions supposedly given by fellow observers. Then, the participants were told that the answers supposedly supplied by their peers were in fact fabrications and given the opportunity to change their answers to the ones they originally gave. The investigators first showed that the participants changed their answers to conform to what they believed to be their peers' beliefs before being told that those answers were fake. Next they showed that strong activation in the amygdala, a relatively more primitive part of the brain associated with emotional memory, was associated with lower likelihood of participants changing their minds back to the truth even when they were informed that the answers provided by their "peers" were fabricated. Strong amygdala activation correlated with strong activation of the hippocampus, an adjacent brain structure that stores memories but was inversely correlated with activity in the PFC.

It is no wonder, then, that conspiracy theorists do not begin addressing their audiences by saying, "I am going to calmly and systematically take you through a series of scientific facts in order to reach a conclusion." Rather, they pack emotional appeals into their presentations, hoping to activate a lot of amygdala-hippocampal memory systems, inhibit audience members' PFCs, and ensure that their message will be resistant to future attempts at reasoned falsification.

It also appears to matter a great deal which emotional appeal you encounter first. Paul Slovic and others have shown that once we are primed to make a decision by an emotional appeal, subsequent appeals, even if they too are emotional in nature, fail to dislodge the first impression. It is almost impossible for us to change our minds, which is troubling, since so much of science advances through the process of dislodging previous ideas.

> These various studies demonstrate that affect is a strong conditioner of preference, regardless of whether the cause of that affect is consciously perceived. They also demonstrate the independence of affect from cognition, indicating that there may be conditions of affective or emotional arousal that do not necessarily require cognitive appraisal.[25]

Subscribing to a conspiracy theory based on the arousal of fear appears to be one such condition.

This difficulty with changing our minds is part of why it is so important for scientists to try to "get there first" when a new conspiracy theory is brewing. For example, a recent study by Brian Hooker, which was retracted by the journal that published it, claimed that the MMR vaccine causes autism in African American children. The Internet immediately exploded with blogs and articles blaming the CDC for "covering up" the "truth." When the study came out, Sara noticed that a Google search of "Hooker autism article" yielded about 10 pages of results before she actually saw a scientific response. The scientists were so far behind the conspiracy theorists that it seemed impossible to believe that anyone would get through all the pages of results in order to ultimately find the scientific information at all.

Another important aspect of the role of affect in the development of conspiracy theories involves memory for the conspiracists' arguments. If we learn something while in an emotionally aroused state, that learned information is stored along with a memory of the emotional state. When the emotional state is then revived, the associated "facts" will also be brought out of memory into consciousness. So, too, whenever the "facts" are even hinted at, the original emotional state is simultaneously revived. Hence, if the conspiracy theorist makes us angry when he tells us a "fact," then by getting us angry again he will also have succeeded in having us remember what he has previously contended to be fact. If we are aroused with anger and fear when we are told that GMOs will somehow do mysterious things to our genes and give us cancer or some other dread disease, the memory of fear and those "facts" are stored in the brain together. Now every time anyone brings up the topic of GMOs, we simultaneously become angry and fearful because the idea that GMOs cause cancer immediately comes to mind. In that frame of mind, any attempt to dissuade us from the idea is rendered nearly impossible because we are in a primitive state of terror. Norbert Schwarz of the Institute for Social Research at the University of Michigan explains:

> When new material is learned, it is associated with the nodes that are active at learning. Accordingly, material acquired while in a particular mood is linked to the respective mood node. When the person is in the same mood later, activation spreads from the mood node along the pathways, increasing the activation of other nodes, which represent the related material. When the activation exceeds a certain threshold, the represented material comes into consciousness.[26]

Some Characteristics of Fictitious Conspiracies

We noted earlier that it would be foolish to debunk all conspiracy claims, since conspiracies *do* occur. So how can we distinguish between a true conspiracy and a false theory? Ted Goertzel lists several factors that may help distinguish true conspiracy theories—like Watergate—from incorrect ones:[27]

- Cascade logic: more and more people are implicated in the cover-up. The number of people ever claimed to be involved in the Watergate scandal was always very small and did not grow over time. False conspiracy theorists must constantly add each new individual who challenges their point of view with scientific data to the list of conspirators.
- Exaggerated claims of the power of the conspirators. In the case of Watergate, there was no need to exaggerate the power of the conspirators—they included the president of the United States. But in a case like the alleged cover-up of vaccines' ability to cause autism, we are asked to believe that drug companies are so powerful that they can keep data secret from hundreds of scientists and government regulators. Maybe drug companies are not so eager to reveal dangers associated with medications they hope to profit from, and maybe the scientists who work for the companies can be dissuaded from revealing those dangers individually, but every bit of data accumulated in drug company studies must be turned over to the U.S. Food and Drug Administration. Also, another government agency, the

Centers for Disease Control and Prevention (CDC), conducts surveillance studies on a host of things that might affect the public health. One such CDC endeavor showed no connection between vaccines and autism. So now we must believe that all of the scientists at two government agencies are in on it. Furthermore, independent scientists at universities all over the world have, without getting funding from drug companies, also reached the conclusion that vaccines don't cause autism. Somehow, all of them must be in on it too. In essence, this massive conspiracy is controlled by super-powerful drug companies that can, even without paying people, control them. As Cass R. Sunstein notes in his book *Conspiracy Theories and Other Dangerous Ideas*, "Conspiracy theorists typically overestimate the competence and discretion of officials and bureaucracies, which are assumed to be capable of devising and carrying out sophisticated secret plans—despite abundant evidence that in open societies, government action does not usually remain secret for very long."[28]

- The lone scientific voice in the wilderness. As we will discuss in more detail in the next chapter, anti-science movements usually have one or more charismatic leaders at their fore and many of them are scientists who want us to believe that they are the victims of a well-organized conspiracy of all the other scientists in his or her field. It is certainly true that groups of scientists often get into feuds with one another over some aspect of the data. In Jack's field, for example, some scientists think that fear is based in a brain structure called the amygdala and other scientists think it is in the bed nucleus of the stria terminalis (BNST). This may seem a ridiculously technical detail (after all, those brain structures are very close to each other in the deepest part of the cortex), but for a while the issue raised considerable passion, with scientists looking for anything they could find to assert that their side was correct. But the idea of getting a large number of scientists together and organizing them into a conspiracy to bully a lone dissenter is a fantasy. The scientists on both sides would surely complain they don't have the travel funds to come to the secret meetings, that there is a grant deadline looming and they don't have the time to join the conspiracy, and that they don't agree with some aspects of the case against the lone dissenter and want changes made in the case against him or her. Peter Duesberg's argument that all of the HIV research community is conspiratorially against him is therefore basically unthinkable—no one could ever get that many scientists to unite around anything other than a huge federal research grant that funded each one of their separate research groups unless it were actually unassailably true and not worth arguing about.

Motive Is Not Enough

What aspects of alleged conspiracies are *not* reliable indicators of an actual plot? We do know that the alleged motive is not enough to prove a conspiracy, but many people fall into the trap of believing that strong incentives are proof of an actual conspiracy. In fact, the perception of a strong motive apparently misleads people into believing that a conspiracy might really exist. In a study conducted at Wabash College in Indiana, Preston R. Bost and colleagues presented research participants with two familiar conspiracy theories (that President Kennedy was not assassinated by a lone gunman and that the U.S. government is concealing aliens in Area 51) and two unfamiliar conspiracy theories (that the Roman emperor Nero burned down Rome in order to justify persecution of Christians and that the Coca-Cola company deliberately introduced a new product with the intent that it fail in order to boost sales of existing products). They found that when the participants considered the familiar conspiracy theories, they tried to use known facts and scientific evidence to evaluate its veracity. However, when evaluating the unfamiliar theories, they mainly relied on the believability of the motives ascribed to the conspirators. That is, if it seemed plausible that the conspirator had a motive, then the conspiracy theory was more likely to be believed. The authors noted, "Even an accumulated body of evidence often consists of elements that are difficult for the layperson to comprehend and remember: statistical probabilities, forensics tests, and complicated paper trails. Motive may provide a simpler cognitive framework within which to evaluate a conspiracy claim."[29]

We can see how this plays out in the debate about foods containing genetically modified organisms (GMOs). Here, the alleged conspiracy is supposedly headed by the giant agricultural company Monsanto and includes government regulators and scientists supposedly on the company's payroll. The scientific issues here are indeed complex, as we discuss in more detail in chapter 5. The overwhelming scientific consensus is that GMOs are not harmful to human health, but the details of how a gene is inserted into the genome of a plant to make it resistant to insects, drought, or herbicides and pesticides requires explaining some complicated genetics. On the other hand, Monsanto is a huge company and its business practices are aimed at bigger and bigger profits. Corporations can and have indeed ignored all kinds of health and safety issues in favor of profits. The tobacco and automobile industries are notorious in this regard. Hence, rather than get into the complexities of genetic modification, we are swayed by the simple belief that Monsanto has a plausible motive to deceive us— that is, a profit motive. We may be able to identify another common thread to the claims of anti-science conspiracy theorists: someone or something is almost always being condemned for making money.

There is no question that people and corporations do a lot of evil things in order to make money. We are now witnessing a panoply of those in the uncovering of what caused the economic recession of 2008. Large financial corporations acted recklessly, with little regard for the security or interest of their clients, in order to make huge profits for their directors. Corporate greed is a real phenomenon, and the battle over how to regulate banks, large manufacturers, and financial institutions without creating unemployment and harming America's cutting edge is apparently not easily resolved.

But the notion that if someone makes money from something then there is automatically something immoral, dangerous, or illegal being done is obviously unhelpful. We are not here debating the ethics of capitalism, the income gap, or free market economies. Rather, we are simply pointing out that it is entirely possible for someone to make a lot of money making a product or providing a service that is useful and safe. That is, it is insufficient to say that because a profit is being made, the result must be evil. Yet this is in general what conspiracy theorists assert, and in doing so they are preying on our feelings of envy and life dissatisfaction rather than arguing science. Just because a drug company makes a lot of money producing vaccines does not mean that vaccines are dangerous. It is true that in order to preserve profits, the drug company has an incentive to cut corners around safety and to cover up problems with its drug, but that does not mean it is doing so. Although we advocate greater disclosure and transparency of the fees doctors and scientists receive from corporations, we do not believe that every, or even most, doctors who get money from drug companies are guilty of misrepresenting the safety and efficacy of medications. Furthermore, conspiracists and the media who give them attention rarely bother to interview the alleged robber barons at the root of the conspiracies.

Reading Michael Specter's article about GMOs in a recent issue of *The New Yorker*, we were surprised to see that he actually did interview and quote an executive of the Monsanto Corporation. In this interview, the executive speaks candidly, admits that Monsanto made some errors (although not covering up any science that disputes the findings that GMOs are safe), and explains why Monsanto believes what it is doing is ethically correct. What is striking to us about this is how rarely it is done.

When a conspiracy theorist uses profits as the basis for the assertion that something is unsafe, be it GMOs, vaccines, ECT, or nuclear power, we must be on guard. Blaming the rich and powerful creates a powerful emotion in those of us who are neither; that resentment quickly escalates into anger, and in a heightened emotional state we are apt to be more vulnerable to false conspiracy theories. It was never necessary to worry about how much money tobacco companies were making in order to prove that cigarette smoking is dangerous. The science was always clear. Therefore, we suggest that an important clue to suspecting a claim of conspiracy to harm our health is the unproven assertion that it must be true because someone is making a profit.

Given the unfamiliarity of the scientific issues involved in something like GMOs, the easiest way for conspiracy theorists to gain popular support is to convince people that Monsanto has a credible motive for dangerous practices. This is a much easier sell than trying to explain genetics and plant biology. As Preston B. Bost and Stephen G. Prunier showed in a study published in 2013, the stronger the supposed motive, the more likely people will believe in a conspiracy.[30] But as anyone who watches police procedural dramas on television knows, there must be a dead body in order for murder to be suspected, not merely a motive to kill someone. By all means, be skeptical about large corporations, governments, professional societies, and the media. Don't believe everything Monsanto, Merck, Pfizer,

R.J. Reynolds, General Motors, Remington, the Food and Drug Administration, or the American Medical Association says. But make sure there is a body before turning a motive into a real crime.

How Should Scientists Respond to the Profit Motive?

At the same time, these results once again make clear the challenge scientists have in correcting our incorrect ideas. As Bost and Prunier conclude,

> If this formulation is correct, it may partially explain why conspiracy theories are resistant to disconfirmation. Skeptics tend to fight conspiracy theories on the battlefield of direct evidence. The merits of this evidence, however, will not change the record of what occurred after the event—where the gains and losses are found—and will therefore not change the perception of motive that can be woven around those gains and losses. And as long as apparent motive remains, so will some of the persuasiveness of the conspiracy theory.[31]

The conspiracy theorists can identify some clear gains and losses. Monsanto, for example, makes a lot of money. So the motive to make money, supposedly by covering up the dangers of GMOs, has led inexorably, in the conspiracists' view, to tremendous financial advantages. Thus, they assert, the conspiracy is proven. Scientists who now come along and try to argue that inserting a gene that makes a canola plant resistant to the lethal effects of glyphosate in Roundup cannot hurt a human being because it is irrelevant to human biology (we aren't weeds) are now addressing an issue that is orthogonal to the conspiracy theorists. That is, the audience for the GMO conspiracy theory is operating along a chain of thought that involves a motive yielding a benefit in order to prove plausibility. In essence, the conspiracists have reframed the issue from one about scientific plausibility to one about the strength of a motive. The only way at this point to attack the conspiracy is to disprove the motive.

For scientists to break this link between motive and outcome they must therefore engage in a two-step process. This will require that they be able to demonstrate unequivocally their independence from whoever is the alleged holder of the motive—in this case, Monsanto. Even though it is far from proven that scientists who received money from Monsanto are guilty of lapses in scientific integrity, in order to get anywhere in combatting distortions of scientific truth the scientist must be able to say, "I know it is entirely possible that Monsanto is a terrible company, run by people who would run over their grandmothers to make a profit. So don't trust a word they say. On the other hand, I have absolutely no connection to Monsanto and I don't profit in any way from GMO foods. I conduct experiments in my laboratory to determine if they are safe, I am an expert in this field, and I have examined all the important scientific studies done in other people's labs. And I am here to tell you that GMOs are safe."

The Isolating Power of the Internet

Because a substantial amount of information about conspiracies is now transmitted via social media, it is time that science proponents learn to use it more effectively. Brian G. Southwell uses the results from a study of attitudes about the vaccine for the H1N1 flu strain to explain how social media works in framing the public's views on healthcare:

> The findings showed that regions of the country where correspondent Twitter messages tended to mention the HINI vaccine in a positive context also tended to have higher flu vaccination rates according to separate US Centers for Disease Control and Prevention data. Regions where sentiment was relatively more negative tended also to have lower flu vaccination rates.... Moreover, the results revealed a distinctly polarized nation with little information flow between well-vaccinated groups and less-vaccinated groups.[32]

Are these two groups of people really so different that there would be no chance of usefully connecting them to each other? In fact, what appears to be going on here is a manifestation of the way that the Internet creates social isolation and polarization.

The Internet has enabled millions of people to connect with one another who otherwise would never have any contact and has broadened our horizons with vast streams of information. But it can also be very isolating and in this way promote adherence to conspiracy theories. Let us take the imaginary example of Cheryl, a well-educated, single mother in her early 40s who is struggling to make ends meet.

She has no time for a social life between working and taking care of two children. She is often lonely but too busy to do anything about it. One night while watching the 10:00 news on television, she sees an interview with a man who takes the position that owning a gun is vital for the protection of home and family. Without disclosing whether he is a member of any political or advocacy group, he tells the story of another man who once thwarted a would-be burglar by shooting the armed invader to death, thus saving his wife and small children who were sleeping in an upstairs bedroom at the time. The man being interviewed is poised with his assault rifle as he declares, "It is guns like this that save our lives from the criminals out there. You cannot wait for the police to come. You need to protect the people you love."

Shaken up, Cheryl goes to her computer and googles the incident about which she has just heard. At the top of the search result list is a link to an organization she has never heard of that seems to have information that corroborates the account of the incident she has just heard. Cheryl clicks on that link, as most of us generally do, because we are under the illusion that what appears first in a Google list is the most reliable. This of course is not true, as Noreena Hertz makes clear:

> We consider most trustworthy those links that appear highest up on Google's search page—the top three results on page 1 of a Google search receive almost 60 per cent of clicks. Yet Google sorts its results on the basis of a website's popularity: in broad terms, the more people who link to the website, the higher up in the results it will be. And popular does not necessarily mean trustworthy. Ideologically charged websites with a high hit rate can easily edge out sound scholarship or truthful testimony.[33]

Looking over the group's website, Cheryl gets even more details, like the names and ages of the children involved in the shooting incident. Their pictures are included. There is a quote from the local sheriff: "Thank goodness we have men like this who fight back against this kind of scum." Reading along, Cheryl learns that there supposedly are many such incidents all over the United States and that they in fact occur on an almost daily basis. "Somewhere in the United States right now," the web page says, "someone is being confronted by an armed madman intent on shooting him. Does he have time to call the police? Or should he take action himself? Those are the questions you need to ask when considering whether to have a gun."

By now Cheryl is pretty sure that this organization is an advocacy group for gun access. She also reads that this group is facing a big challenge: a conspiracy of Eastern liberals, mainstream media, and left-wing politicians are determined to disarm law-abiding citizens and render them helpless against the bands of lawless criminals wandering all over the countryside. Cheryl is asked to click a button, contribute $10, and become a member.

Cheryl has worked a long day and then made dinner, helped with homework, and gotten two children to bed. She is exhausted. She is frightened. Ten dollars seems like a bargain. So she signs up. Not only does she feel like she has done a little something to protect her children, she has joined a group that will send her emails and literature in the regular mail. Maybe she can even go to a meeting once in a while and get out of the house. And she won't feel guilty because this is something she is doing not only for herself but to protect her children and it doesn't cost much.

The important thing to glean from this admittedly dramatized story is that Cheryl has taken no steps to verify anything on the television show or the web page. She has not been given any scientific data or any facts from other sides of the issue. From now on, she will be isolated from every other source of information about guns. Even if she herself does not decide to buy a gun (they are expensive and she wouldn't have the time to learn how to use it), she is now self-identified as a victim of a conspiracy to deny her the right to bear arms, to be safe in her home, and to feel protected from homicidal maniacs who are around every corner. Everyone is out to get her, but there is some safety in joining the one group that sees the issue clearly and will help. As Southwell also notes, "Much of the discussion we seek with others in moments of elevated emotion ... is not necessarily focused on new factual information sharing as much as it is focused on reassurance, coping with stress, and ritualistic bonding."[34] Once again, we see how efforts to counter antiscience conspiracy theories fall short. They are not comforting and do not encourage bonding. Scientists who present the data showing unequivocally that having a gun at home is far more dangerous than protective are not inviting people like Cheryl to join a group. But the isolating power of the Internet ensures that neither pro- nor anti-gun groups talk to each other. Similarly, thinking about the "army of aggrieved parents nationwide who swear vaccines are the reason their children develop autism and who seem impossible to convince otherwise," Chris Mooney and Sheril Kirshenbaum answer a frightening question: "Where do they get their 'science' from? From the Internet, celebrities, other parents, and a few non-mainstream researchers and doctors who continue to challenge the scientific consensus, all of which forms a self-reinforcing echo chamber of misinformation."[35]

In the case of Cheryl, we describe someone who is prone to accepting a conspiracy theory because of her isolation and high level of experienced stress. The situation would be even worse if Cheryl had been reacting to an actual bad event. Neither of Cheryl's children has autism or indeed recently suffered from any significant illness. She is not preoccupied with an accident at a nuclear power plant, is not so depressed that anyone has advised her to get ECT, and does not have a close friend just diagnosed with HIV infection or been held up at gunpoint. Any one of these situations would have made Cheryl even more susceptible to accepting the conspiracy theory. As Sunstein points out, "Terrible events produce outrage, and when people are outraged, they are all the more likely to seek causes that justify their emotional states, and also to attribute those events to intentional action."[36]

Is there a way that we can break this Internet-imposed isolation and at least prevent our friends, our families, and even ourselves from signing on with anti-science conspiracy theory groups in the first place? We do not have an easy answer to that question but stress that most people who become convinced that they are victims of a conspiracy are psychologically normal and not paranoid. Rather, they are people who suffer from low self-esteem, feel powerless, and generally distrust authority.[37] The leader of the conspiracy theory group exploits these characteristics by making the initiate feel welcomed to the group, by emphasizing the us-versus-them aspect of the conspiracy theory, and by ridiculing anything said that contradicts the conspiracy theory. Cass R. Sunstein explains:

> Group leaders may enforce such segregation in order to insulate the rank and file from information that would undermine the leaders' hold on the group. Even if contrary information and arguments are

in some literal sense heard, they will be ridiculed and made a subject of contempt.[38]

As children, all of us got some satisfaction from making fun of people in the "other" group. That is precisely what conspiracy theorists do to make belonging to them feel so socially reinforcing.

Sunstein has advanced a rather radical suggestion to counteract the power of groups on the Internet to spread conspiracy theories: "cognitive infiltration of extremist groups." While acknowledging the ethical problems associated with such an approach, he explains how it might work in the case of conspiracy theories that accuse government agencies of a secret and harmful collusion:

> Hearing only conspiracy accounts of government behavior, [extremist network and group] members become ever more prone to believe and generate such accounts. Perhaps the generation of ever-more-extreme views within these groups can be dampened or reversed by the introduction of cognitive diversity. Government might introduce such diversity—needless to say only under circumstances in which there is a compelling and legitimate need to respond to the conspiracy theory. . . . Under this approach, government agents and their allies might enter foreign chat rooms, online social networks, or even real-space groups and attempt to undermine percolating conspiracy theories by raising doubts about their factual premises, causal logic, or implications for action, political or otherwise.[39]

It is unclear how serious Sunstein is about this suggestion, and it is not one that we feel comfortable endorsing. The last thing we need in fighting conspiracy theories is secretive assaults on websites and chat rooms by government agencies. Even if such activities worked, which is far from likely, scientists would be put in the position of in fact conspiring against the very people they are hoping to educate.

But it may be possible to attempt something like "cognitive infiltration" in a more transparent fashion. The wonderful website Snopes.com is a fun resource for checking out rumors about everything, including health issues. One can choose from many myths that have already been researched. The information provided appears to be systematically collected, unbiased, and largely accurate. It has nice graphics and a kind of breezy style of writing that is engaging. It bursts all kinds of myths, like the one about Typhoid Mary infecting thousands of New Yorkers with typhoid fever or the 2014 study that claimed to invalidate the link between sun exposure and skin cancer. Could there be a way to openly introduce this kind of approach into websites that support anti-science conspiracy theories?

Room for Corrective Action

We began this chapter by bemoaning the difficulty of distinguishing real from fraudulent conspiracy theories. Hopefully, this chapter has suggested both some of the characteristics that can be used to identify anti-science conspiracy theories and consequent approaches to combatting them.

The first principle we wish to emphasize is the need to be on the scene early and vigorously. Research shows that once a conspiracy theory is articulated and circulated it becomes extremely difficult to counteract it. The scientific, medical, and public health communities need to organize an advanced team of intelligence agents, perhaps not unlike those used by the military, to learn of nascent conspiracy theories when they first emerge, to determine whether there is any validity to them, and if there isn't, to begin immediately to marshal efforts to contradict them. Much of this work must be done through sophisticated use of the Internet. Scientists may not have time to become familiar with each new incarnation of social media. They must therefore hire people who do. Fighting a conspiracy theory without using Facebook, Twitter, and Instagram is fruitless. In a few years using those sites will probably have become fruitless as well.

Next, it is important to understand who the proponents of false conspiracy theories generally are. They are characterized by chagrined scientists and doctors who have felt slighted by their colleagues. They often form new organizations with long and provocative names; name themselves the president, director, or CEO; and frequently avoid disclosing how large the membership actually is. Most important, they tend to portray themselves as lone wolves who are the victims of huge and powerful conglomerates usually comprised of some combination of industry, government, and professional societies.

The techniques that these conspiracy theory originators use are also telltale signs of an anti-science position. Motive is emphasized over outcome. Anyone who makes money is automatically criminal. Yet how the conspiracy theorist earns a living is never discussed. The power of the conspiracy is vastly exaggerated. The list of people implicated in the conspiracy grows and grows. Perhaps most important, conspiracy theorists exploit the affective heuristic by couching all of their messages in angry, frightening terms that avoid scientific discourse in favor of high emotion and drama.

It is equally important to understand the profile of people who are most vulnerable to these demagogues. Fundamental to this is recognizing that they are not stupid. They may not have significant scientific sophistication, but they are generally intelligent. They are also usually not psychotic or paranoid. Rather, those who succumb to conspiracy theories tend to be lonely, isolated people who are mistrustful of authority, especially the government, and feel themselves to be under substantial stress. Most important, they feel powerless and are waiting for something to empower them. And indeed, all of us have at times been prone to believing a conspiracy theory.

Besides trying to get there first, scientists and those who care about science must begin now to experiment with different forms of messaging. We simply do not know yet how to balance giving people facts with emotional appeals. How much do we appeal to the amygdala versus the prefrontal cortex? Typically, scientists have not thought of effective education as one of their responsibilities. When pushed to talk to nonscientists, their approach is generally to try to simplify the science. Some are better at this than others, but it may be beside the point because, as we have seen, those who believe in conspiracy theories have been programmed to deny the validity of countervailing data. We need carefully conducted studies to teach us how best to engage with even the most seemingly recalcitrant members of the anti-science population.

Another tricky and for scientists unsettling area to consider when trying to combat false conspiracy theories involves resetting the identification with the victim paradigm. It would be hard to find an actual individual who can demonstrate that her health was harmed by consuming GMO foods. Nevertheless, in this particular conspiracy theory we are asked to feel for those innocent victims who will supposedly be rendered ill because of the conspiracy to put GMOs in what we eat. Similarly, most of us have never been the victims of a home invasion in which armed assailants threatened our lives or the lives of our loved ones. Yet the gun lobby wants us to identify with people who have been or will be such victims. Missing from this scenario is of course the true victims, those victimized by the anti-science conspiracy theorists. These include children starving in Africa because bugs eat the crops they could be eating if GMO seeds had been used; teenagers who shoot themselves with their parents' guns; unvaccinated children who catch measles and develop life-threatening encephalopathies or pass measles on to children being treated for cancer who cannot be vaccinated; people with severe depression who do not respond to psychotherapy or antidepressant drugs and kill themselves when they could have been saved by ECT; and so on. Scientists generally do not give emotion-laden appeals in which these victims are discussed, even though they are real, whereas the conspiracy theorists' "victims" are too often fabrications. Recently, anti-smoking advertisements have become increasingly graphic, showing people with severe pulmonary disease gasping for air. Scientists are more comfortable making statements like "The risk of acquiring chronic obstructive pulmonary disease or COPD is greatly enhanced by cigarette smoking." But as we have seen, that statement does not carry the human, amygdala-provoking, memory-enhancing power that so many of the anti-science statements do. Perhaps it is time to realize that anti-science conspiracy theorists are in fact the conspirators who create real victims. Those victims are the people who actually deserve our empathy, but we know almost nothing about them. Somehow, for example, gun lobbyists have led us to believe that more people are shot to death every year by armed home invaders than by self-inflicted gun wounds. It is time that we learn how to use the power of the Internet, emotional appeals, and compassion for those who feel powerless in order to fight back against the anti-science conspiracy theorists.

Charismatic Leaders

I N THIS CHAPTER, AS IN THE LAST, WE EXPLORE THE WAYS in which skeptical science beliefs are formed in social environments. This time, however, we focus specifically on the leaders of anti-science groups, people we call "charismatic leaders." While behavioral economists and cognitive psychologists have spent much time analyzing the ways in which individual shortcuts and cognitive errors cause irrational beliefs, here we turn to social psychologists to inform us about how being in a group affects the way we process risk, the way we understand complexity, how we decide to whom we give credibility, and how we determine what is true and what is false. We will see that in some cases, people in groups make decisions or hold beliefs that do not resemble decisions or beliefs they would hold on their own. In this way, groups can be said to have transformative capacity. The formation of cooperative groups was foundational in the evolution of the human species. Groups are essential for successful human society. In this chapter, however, we explore the ways in which anti-science groups form around a particular type of leader. Although groups have many important and interesting dynamics, the role of the charismatic leader is a central feature of science denial groups in particular.

We will look at several such charismatic leaders in this chapter: Peter Duesberg, Andrew Wakefield, Jenny McCarthy, Gilles-Éric

Séralini, and Wayne LaPierre. We will also look at the ways in which our brains and minds work in social settings and how exactly we are persuaded. Indeed, some of the features that make us most human, such as our ability to empathize using our imaginations and our desire to be accepted and integrated into social groups—indeed, some of the very things that enable our society to function—are also some of the features that render us most irrational and most prone to the wiles of the charismatic leader.

Leadership Is in the Eye of the Beholder

Before we discuss the figure of the charismatic leader, it is important to examine what factors enable leadership success in the first place. In many ways, leadership is actually created by followers. It is, in some ways, in the eye of the beholder. Leadership theory discusses how people's preconceived notions of how a leader should look and act affect whether certain people rise to the position of "leader." For example, in the business world, someone who is well dressed and outgoing might be immediately labeled as a leader.[1]

Once a group of people has formed a sense of "us," the leader must conform to a leadership *prototype*. That is, the leader must be seen as the epitome of in-group identity. The more the leader is seen as "one of us," the more influence he or she will have.[2] The leader must also be seen as a group "champion." The group must perceive that the leader is in it for the group goal rather than primarily for his or her own benefit.[3] The leader must be proactive about creating the group's identity: he or she should not simply wait for group members to formulate a prototypical leadership role but work hard to create that role, substantiate it in the minds of group members, and ultimately fulfill it.[4] The leader therefore must walk a careful line between being seen as "one of us" and wielding the authority to create and shape the group's identity. An effective leader must take cues from group members but also have control over how the group expresses itself, how it develops, and ultimately what it does and does not support.

What is most striking about this model of leadership is that it is dynamic. Leaders do not exist in a vacuum, and the formation of leaders cannot be viewed as something entirely separate from the formation of groups. That is why this chapter examines both the features of charismatic leaders as well as the theories and science behind group psychology, arguing that the leader and his or her followers go hand in hand. One does not exist without the other, and the psychological features of the group are also key not only to the perception of the leader but also to his or her leadership style. While there has been considerable debate in this field regarding the precise characteristics of the charismatic leader, there has been little debate about the fact that the charismatic leader's authority lies in his or her relationship with followers. Therefore, charisma does not reside exclusively in the leader but more precisely as a relational entity. The interplay between leader and followers is therefore an essential part of the process.[5] The charismatic leader is not fundamentally different from a regular or relatively noncharismatic leader but rather capitalizes more successfully on the particular psychological profile of group membership to create a more intense, perhaps occasionally cult-like, following. The charismatic leader therefore functions more specifically as a persuader.

What Makes a Leader "Charismatic"?

It is also very important for us to state emphatically that we do not categorically equate "charismatic leader" with "demagogue," "snake-oil salesman," or any other negative characterization. Martin Luther King Jr. was a charismatic leader whom we all recognize as one of the most dramatically effective and morally correct people who ever lived. Charismatic leaders can be forces for good, and even those whom we believe distort science and mislead us are often right about some aspects of the issue at hand, although we obviously disagree with the leaders we choose to profile in this chapter. Individuals such as Martin Luther King Jr. and Gandhi used their charisma to instill people with visions of the right way forward and to achieve great and vital societal changes. We simply wish to establish the fundamentals of charismatic leaders as powerful persuaders so that we may better understand what happens when this leadership style is put to work in service of irrational, scientifically incorrect beliefs.

In general, charismatic leaders tend to share the following common characteristics: verbal eloquence, strong communication skills, a potent sense of an "us" versus "them," and a remarkable ability to elicit strong emotions. There is a long-standing debate about whether these abilities are "inborn" or developed and thus whether we all have some capacity to become this type of leader. All leaders must create a sense of "us," but what is perhaps unique about the charismatic leader is that he or she not only creates a much stronger sense of an enemy "them" than any other type of leader but also formulates a sense of "us" that can be so potent that it operates to the exclusion of other identities. That is, the group's "us" becomes so strong that people in the group feel an allegiance to the group identity above all other aspects of their identities. This is certainly true in cults, and we will examine whether some of this strong "us" branding has occurred in some of the health denialist movements under examination in this book.

The concept of the charismatic leader was first formulated by one of the founders of the field of sociology, Max Weber. Weber, who worked in Germany at the end of the 19th and beginning of the 20th centuries, postulated three forms of authority in any society: the charismatic, the traditional, and the rational-legal. According to Weber, charismatic leaders derive their authority from structures outside of the formal legal system and typically derive their legitimacy from their exemplary character. They are therefore often seen as "superhuman" or exhibiting "exceptional powers and qualities."[6] In addition, charismatic leaders are essentially revolutionaries. They often come from the "margins of society" and represent strong breaks with established societal systems.[7] In the 1960s, one scholar identified four characteristics of the charismatic leader: "invocation of important cultural myths by the leader, performance of what are perceived as heroic or extraordinary feats, projection of attributes 'with an uncanny or a powerful aura,' and outstanding rhetorical skills."[8] We will see that many of the charismatic leaders involved in health denialist movements are indeed from "fringe" positions, usually on the fringes of mainstream science. We will also see that most of them have mastered the art of persuasion, exhibit excellent rhetorical skill, and hold themselves up as the exemplars of "true science" in the face of what they perceive as corrupt and self-interested scientific practice.

Cults and Charismatic Leaders

Although cults represent a much more extreme version of the kinds of groups we describe in this book (for instance, we are by no means suggesting that anti-vaccine activists constitute a cult), it is still worthwhile to look at the features of cult leadership and cult formation, because the cult leader is basically the charismatic leader taken to the extreme. In addition, cults are almost always a breeding ground for irrational beliefs, which the leader cultivates and develops in order to keep members in line. Although cults represent a much more extreme version of group formation than anti-vaccine activists or pro-gun activists, it is still helpful to see the charismatic leader in its most extreme form in order to have a thorough understanding of what this figure entails. Sometimes, looking at phenomena in their extreme states gives us the clearest sense of what these phenomena truly are.

Studies of cults as a phenomenon are not scarce. One consistent conclusion of these studies is that cult members are often surprisingly educated, seemingly rational people. In fact, they often possess above-average intelligence, and in many cases are recruited from college campuses.[9] Indoctrination into cults probably occurs in several stages. First is the *softening-up* stage, in which recruits are targeted, invited to meetings, and showered with attention from cult members. In the second stage, *compliance*, recruits begin to experiment with some of the beliefs and behaviors of cult members, even though they may still be skeptical. By the third stage, *internalization*, recruits begin to buy into some of the beliefs of the cult members and find themselves more and more integrated into the group. In the final stage, *consolidation*, recruits become loyal to the cult at all costs.[10] It is this stage that causes some of the tragic effects of cult membership we sometimes see in the news, such as mass shootings or suicides.

Cult leaders are certainly an extreme case, and many exhibit narcissistic features to an unusual, often pathological, degree.[11] Yet some of the characteristics of cult leaders are common among leaders in general and are especially relevant to charismatic leaders. Most strikingly, cult leaders tend to refer to nonbelievers and outsiders explicitly as the "enemy." Charismatic leaders may not be this explicit, but they do create an intense sense of in-group identity that craftily plays on the ways in which group psychology can alter individual needs, preferences, and opinions. Charismatic leaders thus create more of a sense of "us" and "them" than noncharismatic leaders do. In addition, cult leaders are notorious for cutting people off from society, whether this isolation includes removing them physically to a remote area or restricting their contact with family and friends. While charismatic leaders certainly do not all operate with such extreme measures, they do often create an environment in which people become so identified with the ideas of the group that they are impervious to outside influences, including rational and alternative points of view.

How Do Leaders Persuade Us?

Charismatic leaders are essentially persuaders. Nelson Mandela used his charisma to persuade his followers to work to erode apartheid in South Africa. Fidel Castro leveraged his magnetic personality to persuade Cuban citizens to follow and support him during a long period of economic depression and sanctions from important sources of foreign trade and commerce. Aside from being articulate and emotionally savvy, persuaders often have a good sense of the psychological features of group formation and identity. Persuaders also play on known tenets of individual psychology. For example, persuasive messages are often tailored to increase or decrease dissonance in receivers. Persuaders know that people have a strong, intuitive drive to reduce cognitive dissonance, the coexistence in the mind of conflicting ideas.[12] In general, people do not tolerate inconsistency well, and there is also a social drive to appear consistent to others. If a persuader is trying to change an audience's opinions on a particular issue, he or she might seek to arouse dissonance with respect to an opponent's point of view. On the other hand, persuaders might want to reduce the possibility of dissonance by constantly reassuring people that they have made the right choice, that they hold the correct opinion, or that there is no viable reasonable alternative to the action they have taken or what they believe.[13] If persuaders wish to convince people that vaccines are unsafe through a dissonance framework, they might begin by saying: "You all want to keep your children safe and healthy. Doctors and the government have routinely told us that to keep our children safe we must vaccinate them against a host of illnesses. Yet these vaccines are actually causing our children to be sicker than they would otherwise have been without them." This statement creates a sense of dissonance in nearly any caring parent who is not well versed in the scientific and immunological bases of vaccination. The parent will immediately say to him- or herself: "How can I say that I am protecting my child when I am actually exposing her to all of these terrible illnesses by getting her vaccinated?" A sense of internal inconsistency, and hence dissonance, thus arises and the parent will likely do everything he or she can to dissolve this uncomfortable feeling.

In addition, people do not have to devote their full attention to a leader's message in order to be persuaded that it is valid. Psychologists have asserted that there are two routes to persuasion: the central route and the peripheral route. When people scrutinize a message and are persuaded, they are being persuaded via the central route. However, an unscrutinized message may still be persuasive. This is where the peripheral route comes in. In this case, the listener will use various cues, some of which function very much like heuristics, to decide whether to be persuaded. For example, one powerful cue is the number of arguments the persuader uses. In one study, people who knew a lot about a particular topic were completely unpersuaded by a large quantity of weak arguments. People who did not know very much about the topic were very persuaded the more arguments there were, no matter how weak they were.[14] In the case of whether HIV causes AIDS, vaccines cause autism, or GMOs cause cancer, most of us are not able to carefully parse an argument about these complex topics. As a result, we are more likely to be persuaded by heuristic-like "cues," such as the quantity of arguments or the demeanor and authority of the speaker. Flooding the field with an abundance of so-called "studies" and individual cases impresses us. It might be that all of the "studies" are published in minor journals by scientists of questionable credentials and that the cases are cherry-picked rarities that do not represent the majority experience. Nevertheless, a charismatic leader can score points simply by providing a long list.

Charismatic Leaders Appeal to the "Emotional Brain"

To further compound the problem, charismatic leaders almost never speak to our rational sides. Part of what makes them such successful, magnetic leaders is their preference for emotional persuasion. Any CEO knows, and any basic leadership course will teach you, that immediately appealing to people's rational brains will not get you very far. Not only will people not like you but your company will actually not function as well as it would if your employees were encouraged to think emotionally and to see the bigger picture. Rational discourse has an important place in any company, but research shows that leaders are more effective and companies more successful when the emotional brain is prioritized. Followers of charismatic leaders, who operate primarily by speaking to our emotional sides, tend to experience their work as more meaningful, receive higher performance ratings, and work longer hours than those who work for an effective but noncharismatic leader.[15]

Although it is an overly simplistic dichotomy, there is some justification in talking about a "rational" and an "emotional" brain. Neuroscientists note that basic emotions stem from evolutionarily more primitive parts of the brain, particularly the limbic cortex, which includes the amygdala (critical for fear), the insula (necessary for several emotions including fear and disgust), and the nucleus accumbens (the brain's reward center). The sight of a snake activates the amygdala, causing an almost instantaneous set of behavioral and physiological reactions like freezing or fleeing, rapid breathing to increase oxygenation of the muscles, increased heart rate, and increased release of stress hormones like cortisol and adrenaline. Little thought is brought to bear. Show someone a picture of a snake several times, however, and another part of the brain recognizes that this is just a harmless picture and there is no actual danger. That part of the brain is the prefrontal cortex (PFC). Regions of the PFC are designated by location (e.g., ventromedial PFC, dorsolateral PFC) and other names, like anterior cingulate cortex (ACC) and orbitofrontal cortex (OFC). Each has slightly different primary roles in cognition and decision making. In general, the PFC and the limbic cortex turn down the activity of each other. A strongly frightening stimulus activates the amygdala, which inhibits the PFC and permits rapid response. A powerful PFC, on the other hand, can exert reason over the emotional brain. A balance of the two results in the ideal human who can experience deep emotions like love, fear, and compassion but can also read, write, understand mathematics, and plan for the future. Psychiatric illnesses like depression and anxiety disorders seem to involve in part a disruption in the normal connectivity between the PFC and the amygdala; sociopaths appear to have deficient amygdala responses and therefore do not experience normal levels of fear. In this chapter and throughout this book we will often refer to the rational and emotional brains with the understanding that the two are totally interconnected and influence each other in complicated and not always predictable ways.

Jan B. Engelmann of Emory University and colleagues performed an experiment that examined how the brain reacts to the advice of an expert. While having their brain activity imaged and quantified using functional magnetic resonance imaging (fMRI), subjects were asked to make a series of financial decisions; half of the subjects were given expert advice about which choices to make, and the other half were given no advice. As the researchers predicted, the group given the expert advice tended to conform to what the experts told them to do. Perhaps more interestingly, the study showed that neural activity in parts of the brain that are involved in judging probabilities, including the dorsolateral PFC and the cingulate cortex, were blunted among the subjects who received expert advice compared to those who did not. Furthermore, subjects who did go against the advice of the experts showed increased activity in the amygdala, which is associated with fear responses. The authors of the study concluded, "Taken together, these results provide significant support for the hypothesis that one effect of expert advice is to 'offload' the calculation of expected utility from the individual's brain."[16] In other words, the decision-making parts of our brain turn off when experts tell us what to do. Even more important, defying an expert makes us anxious.

At the same time, if a charismatic leader can make us sufficiently frightened when he or she first gives us misleading or false information, it may set in motion neural processes that inhibit our ability to correct this initial impression. In a fascinating experiment by Micah G. Edelson of the Weizmann Institute of Science in Israel and colleagues, subjects' brains were imaged with fMRI when they first received false information and then later were given the correct information. The study first showed that a region in the PFC (anterolateral PFC, alPFC) is activated during what the authors call "recovery from social influence." However, strong amygdala activity during the initial exposure to false information decreased alPFC activity and the ability to correct the initial wrong impression. The study authors concluded,

It is possible that the amygdala activity leads to strongly encoded false memories that dominate the original representations. This in turn may restrict the possibility of recovery. These findings illuminate the process by which errors are, or fail to be, corrected and highlight how social influence restricts subsequent correction, even when that influence is later discredited.[17]

What this means is that when we are told that GMO foods cause cancer, vaccines cause autism, and there are criminals waiting to murder us if we are unarmed, we probably have an intense fear response egged on in part by amygdala activation. When facts are subsequently provided—GMO foods are not harmful to human health, vaccines and autism are unrelated, owning a gun increases the likelihood that the owner will get shot—the amygdala response strongly inhibits the ability of the PFC to correct the influence of the charismatic leaders. Those leaders who are most successful in making us feel frightened also make us most recalcitrant to the evidence that scientific inquiry provides.

Unfortunately, engagement of the emotional brain can sometimes mean neglect of reason and this can be especially problematic when trying to assess cold, hard scientific evidence. This is exactly the effect produced by the charismatic leader—an activated emotional brain and a repressed rational brain. Combining the charismatic style of leadership with topics that require careful scientific investigation and interpretation is precisely the recipe for disaster that fuels health denialist groups. And in fact, there are several reasons to believe that charismatic leadership is particularly suited to anti-science movements. Theorists have suggested that charismatic leadership is critical for organizations that need to induce subordinates to make value judgments and to understand the purpose of the entire movement of the organization. This kind of leadership is much less necessary in organizations that are focused on instrumental matters, such as which technology to use for patient records in a hospital. A lot of charisma is also necessary if compliance with the leader depends heavily on moral judgment and less on material reward.[18] In other words, groups that depend on moral or value judgments require more charismatic leaders to hold subordinates together. This kind of leadership is therefore particularly appropriate for anti-science groups, which, as we have shown, depend not so much on evidence or mechanical facts but instead rely very heavily on emotional appeals and value judgments.

Case Study: Peter Duesberg

In her book on HIV denialism in South Africa, Nicoli Nattrass discusses some striking similarities between the structure of HIV denialist movements and anti-vaccine movements. One of the most significant similarities, Nattrass notes, is the existence in both movements of people she terms "hero scientists." In the case of HIV denialism, these "hero scientists" include figures such as Peter Duesberg, a once well-respected scientist with experience researching retroviruses who brought the supposed debate about the cause of AIDS to a more public sphere. In the case of anti-vaxxers, the main hero scientist is Andrew Wakefield, the author of the retracted 1998 *Lancet* article suggesting a connection between autism and vaccines, who publicized the anti-vaccine position using his position as an authoritative, well-respected scientist. As Nattrass points out, both of these leaders have been skillful users of media, strategically utilizing media channels to create skepticism and to make it seem as though there were a genuine scientific debate going on.[19]

In their book *Merchants of Doubt*, Naomi Oreskes and Erik M. Conway profile some of the "hero scientists" and reveal a consistent pattern: a once distinguished scientist with outstanding academic credentials seems at some point to go astray, adopting fringe ideas and portraying himself as a victim of the very establishment in which he was once a major leader. For example, one of the leaders of the tobacco industry cover-up of the carcinogenicity of cigarettes was Frederick Seitz:

> Seitz was one of America's most distinguished scientists. A wunderkind who had helped to build the atomic bomb. Seitz had spent his career at the highest levels of American science: a science advisor to NATO in the 1950s; president of the National Academy of Science in the 1960s; president of Rockefeller University . . . in the 1970s.[20]

Because of his distinguished past, Seitz was able to garner the attention of both the media and Congress and his defense of nicotine was taken seriously in those circles for decades.

Duesberg was similarly preeminent in the scientific world. A PhD in chemistry, he gained international acclaim in the 1970s for his groundbreaking work in cancer research. In 1986, at the young age of 49, he was elected to the National Academy of Sciences and also received an Outstanding Investigator Award from the U.S. National Institutes of Health (NIH). He was widely considered a scientist of great importance worldwide. Yet starting in the late 1980s, Duesberg began publishing articles and eventually a book, called *Inventing the AIDS Virus*, in which he claimed that the human immunodeficiency virus (HIV) is not the cause of AIDS and proffered multiple conspiracy theories to explain why the scientific establishment disagreed.

In many ways, Duesberg can be regarded as the father of the AIDS denialist movement. The movement reached its most tragic peak with the public denialist stance of South African president Thabo Mbeki, who served from 1999 to 2008, but Duesberg began publishing his theories as early as 1987. Duesberg's ideas had their greatest influence when he sat on Mbeki's Presidential Advisory Panel on HIV and AIDS in 2000. Ever since then, Duesberg has been looked to as the "hero scientist" of the HIV/AIDS denialist movement.

One strategy Duesberg has on his side is simply volume. He has published a 500-page book arguing that the HIV/AIDS epidemic is basically a myth created by greedy virologists; he has also continued to write prolifically on the subject in every venue that will still have him. Most reputable scientific journals now refuse to publish Duesberg's work, so he has switched to bombarding fringe journals, Internet sources, and popular media with his theories. His most recent 2014 article on the subject was published in the *Italian Journal of Anatomy and Embryology*.[21] As noted earlier in this chapter, the peripheral route of persuasion often relies on the mere volume of arguments proffered. Duesberg's prolific publishing and long-winded book reveal an interest in appealing to this form of persuasion.

One of Duesberg's most potent strategies, however, is to present his side of the argument as something that people really value: scarce information. Duesberg repeatedly makes it seem as though he is giving his readers "inside" information that is precious and generally unavailable. For example, he draws a long analogy between the supposed "cover-up" of the "fact" that HIV does not cause AIDS and the SMON incident in 1960s Japan. For a long time, SMON (subacute myelo-optic neuropathy), a condition causing paralysis, blindness, and sometimes death, was thought by scientists to be caused by a virus. Eventually, however, they discovered that SMON was really caused by the drug clioquinol, commonly used as prophylaxis for traveler's diarrhea. Duesberg uses faulty logic to "demonstrate" that this occurrence must be the same thing that is going on with HIV/AIDS, that AIDS is really caused by toxic antiretroviral drugs, that HIV has nothing to do with it, and that scientists are harping on the viral "hypothesis" in order to keep virology, a dead field in Duesberg's opinion, alive. He draws inappropriate comparisons between the SMON case and the discovery of HIV as the cause of AIDS in order to suggest that the same "mistake" must be going on with AIDS.

The troubling logical errors embedded in these comparisons aside, Duesberg uses a very powerful rhetorical and persuasive strategy in telling the SMON story. He makes the reader feel as though this information, presumably kept relatively quiet by the U.S. government, is a well-kept secret and access to it is scarce. Duesberg therefore offers his readers an inside glance at a source of information that would otherwise be unavailable to them. Before making a sweeping comparison between SMON and the HIV/AIDS epidemic, Duesberg notes, "Once the truth about SMON could no longer be ignored, the episode dissolved into lawsuits for the thousands of remaining victims. This story has remained untold outside of Japan, ignored as being too embarrassing for the virus hunters. It deserves to be told in full here."[22] By making this statement, Duesberg essentially tells his readers: "Here is some juicy, private information that has been kept from you for a long time, and I am finally going to make it available to you."

When people feel that a piece of information is scarce or difficult to obtain, they tend to feel more persuaded by it. This phenomenon has been well established in the realm of material goods: scarce items generally sell for higher values in the free market, reflecting the way in which people value scarcity. More recently, psychologists have begun to test whether the same is true about less tangible items, such as information. One experiment illustrates the principle quite well. The owner of a beef-importing company called the company's customers, buyers for supermarkets and retail food outlets, to ask them to purchase beef under three different conditions. One group simply heard a standard sales presentation. A second group heard the sales presentation and were told that beef would soon be in short supply. A third group heard the sales presentation, were told that beef would soon be in short supply, and were also told that the information that the beef would soon be in short supply was exclusive information that no one else but them knew. The second group bought the same amount of beef as the first group. However, the third group, who were led to believe that they had been privileged with the "exclusive" news that the beef supply would soon run short, purchased six times as much beef as the first group.[23] The results of this experiment suggest the strong effects not only of commodity scarcity but also of the illusion of information scarcity on people's ability to be persuaded.

Like cult leaders, Duesberg also creates an extremely strong sense of "them" to pit the "us" against. This strong formulation of group identity has a significant ability to alter the way we think about things that are as straightforward as the probability of a particular event happening to us. Strong group membership can distort even a number that seems immune to manipulation. Duesberg achieves this primarily by making mainstream science look like a relentless form of consensus culture:

> Few scientists are any longer willing to question, even privately, the consensus views in any field whatsoever. The successful researcher— the one who receives the biggest grants, the best career positions, the most prestigious prizes, the greatest number of published papers—is the one who generates the most data and the least controversy. The transition from small to big to mega-science has created an establishment of skilled technicians but mediocre scientists, who have abandoned real scientific interpretation and who even equate their experiments with science itself.[24]

Duesberg here constructs a new view of the scientific world: a consensus culture in which all the revered and established researchers operate simply as individual replicas of some dogmatically accepted central truth. By minimizing the intense kind of conflict, disagreement, and rigorous debate that actually goes on in the scientific community, Duesberg makes the "enemy" look much more unified than it actually is. Unifying the enemy ultimately functions as a strategy to then unify the opposition. This is in fact a favorite strategy of charismatic leaders, and it has a significant effect on people's ability to parse the information that is truly coming from the "other side." Once the "enemy" has been consolidated, followers of the charismatic leader have much less access to the individual arguments of those in the opposing camp and have lost the ability to analyze information from these camps unfiltered by the leader.

Duesberg is often cited as a forefather of the HIV denialist movement, and his idea that HIV does not cause AIDS but instead is really caused by illegal drug abuse and antiretroviral medication, which functions as a central tenet of the HIV denialist movement, has even been termed the "Duesberg hypothesis." Look at any HIV denialist website, paper, book, or video and all will cite Duesberg as a major figure in the formation of the movement. He therefore earns the title of a movement leader. Beyond that, we are arguing that he is in fact a "charismatic leader," due to the rhetorical tactics he has used, the popularity of his ideas among HIV denialists, and the way in which he has been worshipped and given undue amounts of authority by this group of denialists. In order to understand HIV denialism, it is essential to understand the charismatic leaders in front of the movement. In a similar manner, in order to understand the anti-vaccine movement, it is vital to understand the charismatic leaders at its helm. Without this kind of understanding, our view of these movements is by definition incomplete.

Case Study: Andrew Wakefield

Ever since he published a paper claiming a link between vaccines and autism in *The Lancet* in 1998, Andrew Wakefield has been a major champion of the anti-vaccine movement, frequently speaking at their rallies and conferences. Like Peter Duesberg, Andrew Wakefield had a distinguished background as a well-respected gastroenterologist and medical researcher. When it was uncovered in 2010 that Wakefield had been accepting money from a defense lawyer to publish certain findings, *The Lancet* paper was retracted and Wakefield eventually lost his medical license. In addition to obvious conflicts of interest, the paper was scientifically unsound, with only 12 nonrandomly selected subjects and no comparison group.[25] Nevertheless, a strong contingent, including Wakefield himself, has persisted in the belief that his findings are in fact the scientific truth and that his demise is the product of a conspiracy propagated mostly by the medical community's slavish deference to the pharmaceutical manufacturers of vaccines. This is, of course, the type of conspiracy theory we discussed in chapter 1.

Wakefield has many of the characteristics of a strong charismatic leader, and these characteristics have served him well as *the* "scientific" spokesman for the anti-vaccine movement. If Jenny McCarthy represents the "human," parental perspective of the movement, Wakefield is supposedly the science behind it. Wakefield's method is to characterize himself as a victim while emphasizing the desperate, inquisitional strategy of the opposition, which consists of the public health community, the American Academy of Pediatrics, and the pharmaceutical industry. In an interview with Anderson Cooper on CNN, Wakefield refers to the journalist who exposed him, Brian Deer, as a "hit man" who was being paid by some unidentified "them." He calls the retraction of his paper by *The Lancet* and his condemnation by the British General Medical Council a "ruthless pragmatic attempt" to cover up his own sincere investigation of vaccine damage. In an interview with Robert Scott Bell, Wakefield refers to the medical community as a "religion" that no one is allowed to question and calls the allegations against him an "attack."[26] And during the American Rally for Personal Rights, at which Wakefield was the keynote speaker, he proclaimed that the allegations against him were "a futile public relations exercise that will fail."[27] These examples show Wakefield expending quite a bit of energy crafting an identity for his ruthless, calculating enemies. As we have seen, the creation of a strong enemy is a common tactic of charismatic leaders that helps solidify the group identity of his followers.

Wakefield also does an effective job of justifying the need for a charismatic leader in the first place. He frames the situation as a battle between the interests of the patients and the interests of the public health community and pharmaceutical industry. He suggests that the moment is ripe for a "social revolution," embodying the charismatic leader's position on the fringes of mainstream society as an instigator of revolution, as originally identified by Weber. Like the head of the National Rifle Association, Wayne LaPierre, Wakefield broadens the playing field from one limited to a specific issue—vaccines or guns—to a much larger issue of personal rights and freedom. He calls autism a "worldwide pandemic" and refers to vaccines as an "environmental catastrophe." The choice is simple, he asserts: we can either attend to our patients or walk away. The scientific community must choose between "fidelity and collusion," he proclaims. And parents must demand the right to choose "for the sake of the future of this country and the world." All of this rhetoric effectively establishes Andrew Wakefield as a charismatic leader. A victim of the status quo, Wakefield has suffered the consequences of choosing the correct path and has lost his medical license, his research position, his reputation, and, he says, even his country. Yet all of this, he claims, is nothing compared to the suffering of parents of children with autism and other developmental disorders. Like the true charismatic leader, he demonstrates that his overwhelming commitment to the cause is so strong that he was willing to lose not only his license but also his home. He further emphasizes his commitment to the cause through an elaborate process of self-effacement, in which he calls himself "irrelevant," stating: "It doesn't matter what happens to me. It is a smokescreen."[28] The real issue here is not his career or his reputation but the pure goal of saving the children. Wakefield speaks with the language of a religious zealot. He does not talk science—even he has been unable to replicate his "findings" in a separate experiment. Everything he says rests on 12 children, some of whom did not actually have autism and others who had it before they received the MMR vaccinations.[29] In retrospect, there is absolutely no science involved here.

Wakefield is certainly a powerful communicator, with a great deal of verbal eloquence, strategic use of hand gestures and facial expressions for maximum animation, and the ability to create a sense of urgency. Wakefield's ability to persuade lies largely in his charismatic qualities, especially his ability to unify "us" against "them" and to invent a crisis that requires immediate action and the guidance of a cast-out, self-sacrificing, superman leader. Moreover, Wakefield is the face of empathy standing in opposition to a harsh scientific and medical world that supposedly panders to the whims of the pharmaceutical industry. Wakefield's goal is to protect the children and to grant parents their freedom to choose, and he makes very clear that he is willing to sacrifice everything to achieve this goal. In his self-sacrifice, his call to revolution, and his existence on the fringes of mainstream science, Wakefield embodies the charismatic leader and all of the psychological consequences that accompany this figure.

Case Study: Jenny McCarthy

Jenny McCarthy may not seem like the most obvious choice here, since she does not have the credentials of a scientist such as Peter

Duesberg or Andrew Wakefield. Nonetheless, she is a major leader of the anti-vaccine movement, and there are reasons to believe that her style is indeed charismatic. First of all, she is to some physically attractive. This feature helps her get attention. Watching a few of McCarthy's media appearances and her rallies in places such as Washington, DC, we can see that she embodies many of the features of charismatic leaders. Her tone of voice is engaging and captivating. Her facial expressions are animated. She makes direct, sustained eye contact. She is expressive with her hands, and she even smiles and laughs as she finds appropriate in order to draw her audience toward her.[30] She is certainly extraverted, which leadership theorists have maintained is a particularly charismatic feature for female leaders.[31]

We need not look much further than McCarthy's speech at the 2008 "Green Our Vaccines" rally in Washington, DC, to see many of these principles at play. For one thing, videos of the rally show an enamored crowd chanting McCarthy's name as she takes her place at the podium. This kind of devotion to a leader suggests a charismatic leadership style, in which the leader is viewed as someone with special powers and as someone to be admired as a superhero. The sound of "Jenny! Jenny!" being shouted in unison is certainly a striking one, and it already indicates, before McCarthy even starts speaking, that she at least has the kind of following that a charismatic leader must attract.

Once she starts speaking, McCarthy employs a whole host of charismatic leader strategies, many of which are designed to stimulate emotional responses in her followers. As we noted earlier, a movement designed to reinforce a certain point of view—one that is based not in facts but in "values" that supposedly promote caring for our children and taking their health into our own hands—is particularly prone to the skills of charismatic leaders. The leader in this type of situation can make all the difference, as opposed to one involving a group deciding on something more mundane and mechanical. McCarthy begins by insisting that everyone in the crowd come closer to the podium. She takes multiple strategic pauses and speaks in a kind of storytelling voice with extreme animation and constant fluctuations in her tone. She exhorts parents to be empowered and to take the safety of their children into their own hands. She refers to her audience multiple times as "you guys" and encourages everyone to show pictures of their children to the media cameras at the rally. Finally, she calls this a time in history for citizens to change the world and to fight the powers that be.[32] Once again, and like many charismatic leaders, she broadens the scope of the appeal beyond the main issue to one that involves universal concepts of justice and freedom, things with which almost no one disagrees. Thus, the audience gets confused—is it really focused on the cause of autism or on freedom and justice for all? Any hint at science is notably absent from the discourse.

In this short speech, McCarthy displays many signs of charismatic leadership. By drawing the crowd closer to her, she creates an even stronger sense of "us," inviting her followers in to create a more unified group. Similarly, by referring to her followers as "you guys," she creates a sense of unity among them to fight against the opposition. One can almost visualize the outpouring of oxytocin from the hypothalamus of every person in attendance, making them all feel loved and secure.[33] Her tone of voice and strategic, dramatic pauses draw listeners in and resemble the kind of sustained eye contact and animation that are often identified as central features of the charismatic leader's style. Perhaps most interesting, in closing her speech, McCarthy calls upon her followers to embrace this as a time in history when citizens can rise up, change the world, and fight the powers in charge. As discussed earlier in this chapter, Max Weber defined the charismatic leader as someone who takes charge from the fringes and leads followers through a form of revolution. Here, McCarthy takes advantage of this formulation and specifically crafts the movement as a revolution of sorts. She encourages her followers to view this as an opportunity to challenge and perhaps overthrow those in power and to embrace this admittedly fringe view as a chance to change the world. This kind of revolutionary language is certainly in line with the prerogatives of the charismatic leader.

Although Jenny McCarthy may lack the scientific training of an Andrew Wakefield or Peter Duesberg, she does have many of the features of a charismatic leader that, as we have shown, create a very specific dynamic with her followers. Understanding the anti-vaccine movement is therefore dependent on understanding how precisely these leaders lead and the psychology involved in responses to different types of leadership.

Case Study: Gilles-Eric Séralini

The trailer to the documentary *Tous Cobayes Fa Anglais* begins with a startling claim: after the atomic bomb was dropped on Hiroshima at the end of the Second World War the U.S. Department of Energy had a lot of money and staff and did not know what to do with them, so the agency decided to embark on the genome sequencing project, which led directly to nuclear energy and genetically modified organisms (GMOs).[34]

You can view this trailer on the website GMOSeralini, a very attractively designed website that represents the ideas of its founder, French scientist Gilles-Eric Séralini. Séralini is the darling of the anti-GMO movement. Like Duesberg and Wakefield, his résumé is very impressive. Since 1991 he has been professor of molecular biology at the University of Caen. His earlier work was in endocrinology, and his lab produced important findings about an enzyme called aromatase that were published in fairly high level journals. It may be the fact that this enzyme is involved in an herbicide called glyphosate, discovered and marketed by the Monsanto Corporation under the trade name Roundup, that attracted Séralini's interest, but for whatever reason he turned his attention away from endocrinology to testing GMOs in rats. In 1997 he began advocating for a moratorium on GMO foods. He also formed the Committee for Research and Independent Information on Genetic Engineering (CRIIGEN), an advocacy organization that supports legislation to regulate GMOs in foods.

To understand Séralini's brand of charismatic leadership, it is useful to know a bit about the anti-GMO movement. The battle against GMOs, which has been waged for 2 decades, is absolutely fascinating for anyone trying to comprehend the roots of science denial. There is actually no direct evidence that anyone has ever been harmed by eating food that contains genetically modified ingredients, and we have been consuming them for a very long time—centuries, in fact, from one vantage point. Nevertheless, individuals and groups have risen up passionately condemning them, demanding they be banned or at the very least that foods containing them be so labeled.

Vermont was the first state to pass a law mandating labeling food that contains GMOs. Somehow, opposing GMOs has become a left-wing cause. Whole Foods refuses to stock them, and Greenpeace demands their abolition. But as a graphic in *The Economist* noted, there are 3.1 million deaths in the world every year from malnutrition and 0 deaths every year from genetically modified food. *The Economist* article concludes, "The outlook is unappetising. Food scares are easy to start but hard to stop. GMO opponents, like climate-change deniers, are deaf to evidence. And the world's hungry people can't vote in Vermont."[35] In Hawaii, a debate about GMOs brought out advocates on both sides, but as *New York Times* reporter Amy Harmon observed, "Popular opinion masqueraded convincingly as science, and the science itself was hard to grasp. People who spoke as experts lacked credentials, and G.M.O. critics discounted those with credentials as being pawns of biotechnology companies."[36]

Into this fray emerged a charismatic leader. Gilles-Eric Séralini became famous—some would say infamous—in 2012 with the publication of his paper "Long Term Toxicity of a Roundup Herbicide and a Roundup-Tolerant Genetically Modified Maize" in the journal *Food and Chemical Toxicology.*[37]

In the study, Séralini and his colleagues at Caen fed rats for 2 years with Monsanto's Roundup and Roundup Ready corn (formally known as glyphosate-resistant NK603 maize). They reported that compared to control rats not given the herbicide or the GMO corn, those fed Roundup and Roundup Ready developed more tumors, had liver and kidney abnormalities, and died sooner. The conclusion in the abstract reads, "These results can be explained by the non linear endocrine-disrupting effects of roundup, but also by the overexpression of the transgene in the GMO and its metabolic consequences." Not exactly easy reading for the nonspecialist, but essentially asserting that the two products damaged the rodents' hormonal and metabolic systems. Séralini introduced the paper at a press conference of select journalists who were required to sign a confidentiality agreement prohibiting them from discussing the study with other scientists. This unusual maneuver prevented consenting journalists from obtaining any comments from independent scientists. Furthermore, at the press conference Séralini introduced his new book, *OGM, le vrai débat* (GM foods, the real debate), and a film about the study. Séralini appeared to be on an aggressive public relations adventure, not something scientists commonly get into when they publish a paper in a scientific journal.

The paper won immediate praise and dire warnings from anti-GMO organizations. The European Commission ordered the European

Food Safety Agency (EFSA) in Parma, Italy, to evaluate it, and both Russia and Kenya put bans on GMOs.

Yet even more robust was the wave of derision the paper received from scientists. Just reading the abstract conclusion quoted in the previous paragraph gives an immediate hint that there might be a problem. What Séralini et al. did was an association study in which they claim to have observed a relationship between consuming GMO corn and getting tumors. But the wording of the abstract implies that they found a biological basis for this supposed association, what they call "metabolic consequences." In fact, no such biology was discovered in the study or reported in the paper. Indeed, it is hard to understand what plausible biology could link a gene for herbicide resistance to all of these effects. While again the scientific details behind that assertion are complex, what we are pointing out is the gene put into Roundup Ready to make it resistant to the herbicide Roundup should not be able to affect any other system, including a rat's metabolism. If it does, then a lot more data and explanation would have had to be included in the paper to demonstrate the claim.

But more important, a host of scientists immediately noticed all kinds of problems with the way the study was designed and analyzed. There were clearly too few rats, the strain of rats used is notorious for developing spontaneous tumors at a high rate, and unusual statistics were employed, leading to widespread insistence that the study could not possibly have found any actual link between the GMO and the tumors. In 2012, after Séralini refused to withdraw it, the journal announced it was retracting the paper. The retraction notice reads,

> A more in-depth look at the raw data revealed that no definitive conclusions can be reached with this small sample size regarding the role of either NK603 or glyphosate in regards to overall mortality or tumor incidence. Given the known high incidence of tumors in the Sprague-Dawley rat, normal variability cannot be excluded as the cause of the higher mortality and incidence observed in the treated groups.... Ultimately, the results presented ... are inconclusive.[38]

Séralini and his colleagues of course protested the retraction, accusing the journal of "double standards," and defended the study.[39] They also noted that they had sued Monsanto and won the right in court to see raw data from the company's studies, which had been claimed to show no such harm from Roundup Ready. On the contrary, Séralini stated, his analysis of the data confirmed that the company had obscured harmful effects.

Now that the battle was on, Séralini became a self-declared victim of Monsanto and the scientific establishment. In video interviews he is an impassioned orator who declares himself in favor of "food democracy" and "transparency." He decries that pesticides are "inside GMOs" and fighting this "should be a matter of revolution."[40] Note once again the appeal to revolution used also by the other charismatic leaders discussed in this chapter and identified by Weber as integral to charismatic leadership. In an interview on the Internet he said, "It is the same problem as mad cow disease" and "GMOs can be used to make war, and there are two methods—the soft one and the tough one."[41] Séralini now has all the credentials of a charismatic leader of an anti-science group. He has a legitimate scientific résumé, he has crafted himself as the victim of imperious and malevolent forces that threaten our right to choice and safety, and he has broadened the agenda to encompass such widespread ills as nuclear holocaust and war. He delivers a powerful message on the Internet, in books, and in documentary films. His science is highly suspect, but his abilities as a speaker and persuader are nonpareil.

Against this charisma, will anyone heed the words of the following editorial written by scientists in 2013?

> New technologies often evoke rumors of hazard. These generally fade with time, when, as in this case, no real hazards emerge. But the anti-GMO fever still burns brightly, fanned by electronic gossip and well-organized fear-mongering that profits some individuals and organizations. We, and the thousands of other scientists who have signed the statement of protest, stand together in staunch opposition to the violent destruction of [work testing] valuable advances such as Golden Rice that have the potential to save millions of impoverished fellow humans from needless suffering and death.[42]

Case Study: Wayne LaPierre

There are statements that Wayne LaPierre, executive vice-president and CEO of the 5-million-strong National Rifle Association (NRA), makes with which almost no one could disagree.

"Freedom has never needed our defense more than now."

"We're worried about the economic crisis choking our budgets and shrinking our retirement. We're worried about providing decent healthcare and a college education for our children. We fear for the safety of our families—it's why neighborhood streets that were once filled with bicycles and skateboards, laughter in the air, now sit empty and silent."

"Political dishonesty and media dishonesty have linked together, joined forces, to misinform and deceive the American public. Let's be straight about it—the political and media elites are lying to us."[43]

We have taken these comments from LaPierre's 2014 address to the Conservative Political Action Conference out of context to make a point about charismatic leaders: one of their signatures is to take whatever issue with which they are involved and turn it into something that shakes every aspect of our fundamental existence. Notice that both left-wing and right-wing activists would likely agree with all of these statements: everyone is concerned with incursions on our freedom, the economy, healthcare, and declining urban areas.

One can easily imagine an advocate for almost any cause articulating the same sentiments as those of LaPierre. We have already pointed to Séralini's assertion that GMOs are an assault on our freedom. A corrupt media that refuses to recognize the truth is the mantra of almost every activist who sees him- or herself as a victim. In this case, we can insert the notion that the solution to all of these problems is owning a gun and we have LaPierre's version. With remarkably little effort, one could replace all references to guns in his speech with mentions of any other cause, say rights for LGBT people—a cause one doubts LaPierre has much enthusiasm for—and the piece would work as well in arousing us to gross injustice and personal danger. Thus, LaPierre, like many charismatic leaders, actually distracts us from the specific issue at hand—in this case, the wisdom of personal gun ownership—and moves us to a world of platitudes and universal concerns that rouse our emotions without taxing our analytical skills.

Born in 1949, Wayne LaPierre received an undergraduate degree at Sienna College and a master's degree from Boston College. He began working for the NRA in 1977 and in 1991 he became its head. According to the Educational Fund to End Gun Violence, he is paid about $1 million a year by the NRA. It is difficult to find accurate biographical information about him on the Internet, which lends an aura of mystery to him. Several sites claim that he was deferred from military service during the Vietnam War because of an emotional condition, which would be ironic given his insistence that gun violence is entirely the result of untreated mental illness, but these are mostly sites that are antagonistic to the NRA and it is difficult to verify the information.[44]

Whether or not LaPierre did have emotional problems that kept him out of the army, he and the NRA have latched onto mental illness as one of their key rallying cries for the basis of gun violence. The problem is not, he repeatedly tells us, people having guns; rather, it is only mentally ill people having guns about which we should worry. His solution is to make sure the mentally ill are prevented from owning guns. LaPierre and the NRA insist that this will solve the gun violence problem and leave the bulk of the population who do not suffer from mental illness free to enjoy their weapons in peace.

Many people have the notion that "crazy" people are dangerous. Put a gun in the hands of someone with mental illness and a murder is likely to happen, they think. As Heather Stuart noted in an article in the journal *World Psychiatry*, "Indeed, the global reach of news ensures that the viewing public will have a steady diet of real-life violence linked to mental illness."[45] In a recent survey, most respondents favored requiring states to report to a national gun control database the names of all people who have either been involuntarily committed to a hospital for psychiatric treatment or been declared mentally incompetent by a court.[46] In general, the one type of gun control legislation that most people support is the variety that restricts seriously mentally ill people from possessing firearms.

While we do not think there is anything necessarily wrong with preventing people with serious mental illness from having guns, it is not a solution to gun violence for at least two reasons:

1. Most gun homicides are committed by people who do not have mental illness.
2. If one could stop mentally ill people from owning guns it might reduce the suicide rate but would have almost no impact on the homicide rate.

The mass of available data concerning the propensity to shoot a human being instead of a hunted animal does not make for easy reading. It involves complicated statistical analyses of data collected from large populations. Because no one can do a randomized clinical trial and control for all of the confounding variables involved in who does or doesn't own a gun, figuring out who it is that shoots people mandates some very messy experimental designs and fancy mathematical tests. This situation is made all the more difficult by a law our Congress passed that forbids the CDC from conducting research on gun violence. These are generally not the kinds of things that charismatic leaders want to delve into; LaPierre prefers basing his arguments on "facts" like these he laid out in a 2014 speech:

> There are terrorists and home invaders and drug cartels and carjackers and knockout gamers and rapers, haters, campus killers, airport killers, shopping mall killers, road-rage killers, and killers who scheme to destroy our country with massive storms of violence against our power grids, or vicious waves of chemicals or disease that could collapse the society that sustains us all.[47]

If LaPierre were really interested in the data, some of it actually at first seems to support his position: recent data do support the popular belief that people with some forms of mental illness are more likely than the general population to commit violent acts. These tend to be people with psychotic illnesses who suffer from paranoid delusions.[48] One recent study showed that delusions of persecution, being spied on, and conspiracy were linked to violent acts, but only when the perpetrator is especially angry, such as during an argument.[49] These kinds of delusions can make the person feel threatened to the point of believing there is a need for a violent defense. Delusional people tend to have the paranoid form of schizophrenia, suffer from bipolar disorder and be in the midst of psychotic manic episodes, or be intoxicated with stimulant drugs like amphetamines and cocaine.

But that is only the first part of the story, which becomes considerably more complicated and at the same time interesting. First, even given that a segment of the population of people with mental illness is statistically more likely to commit violent acts than the general population, the fact remains that mass murders by mentally ill people are rare events—too rare, experts agree, to be predictable.[50] Newtown was a great tragedy, but it accounted for only 26 of the approximately 10,000 people who were killed in gun homicides in 2012. It is unlikely, for example, that any mental illness registry would have identified the shooter in Newtown. In fact, only 3–5% of violent acts are committed by people with mental illness, and most of these do not involve guns.[51] The American Psychiatric Association has pointed out that the vast majority of people who commit violent acts are not mentally ill.[52] When mentally ill people do commit violent acts, they usually do so in the context of an interpersonal conflict, not a well-planned mass murder.[53]

There is one form of mental illness that is clearly associated with an increased risk of violence and should be attracting much more of LaPierre and the NRA's attention: alcohol and drug abuse. Studies have repeatedly shown that drinking significantly increases the chance that a person will commit a violent act.[54] Neighborhoods with a high density of liquor stores have higher rates of violence than those with fewer liquor stores.[55] Alarmingly, people who own guns are more likely than non–gun owners to binge-drink, drink and drive, and to be heavy drinkers.[56] Heavy alcohol use is particularly common among people who carry guns for protection. Alcohol is also well known to be a significant factor in many cases of suicide by firearm.[57] As an editorial in *The New York Times* pointed out,

> Focusing on the mentally ill ... overlooks people who are at demonstrably increased risk of committing violent crimes but are not barred by federal law from buying and having guns. These would include people who have been convicted of violent misdemeanors including assaults, and those who are alcohol abusers.[58]

Given all of these data, why does Wayne LaPierre continue to focus on the issue of mental illness as the root of all gun violence? After all, the Second Amendment, which he holds to be so precious, does *not* say "The right of the people—*except the ones with a psychiatric diagnosis*—to keep and bear Arms, shall not be infringed." Why wouldn't this kind of restriction also represent a "slippery slope" to LaPierre, the first step toward taking everyone's guns away?

Clearly, LaPierre's inflexible support of the Second Amendment is not, in fact, absolute. This is characteristic of charismatic leaders—the designation of an "out" group as the enemy. Rightly or wrongly, LaPierre senses that the mentally ill are not a sympathetic group to most Americans and therefore he does not see any risk in branding them as the true source of the problem. It is not guns or people who own guns that we need to worry about, he tells us: it is "crazy" people. Organizations like the National Alliance on Mental Illness (NAMI) struggle to defend the rights of people with psychiatric illness and to point to the data demonstrating that this population is, in fact, a very minor contributor to the problem of gun violence in the United States. But data are not LaPierre's forte. He has crafted a potent tool of blaming journalists and liberals for attempting to violate a basic American right and thereby dooming us to face, unarmed, criminals, terrorists, and the mentally ill. Having frightened us, he can then drive home his point with statements like "The political elites can't escape and the darlings of the liberal media can't change the God-given right of good people to protect themselves."[59]

Like all of the charismatic leaders we have profiled, LaPierre does not try to convince us with data or facts of any kind. He could cite some studies that support his point of view, even if they are in the minority among scientific reports and not given credence by the majority. But instead he scares us and then tells us we are on the side of freedom, God, and our children if we do what he says. For many people, these are hard arguments to resist.

What Links Charismatic Leaders?

Can we identify any patterns that link these charismatic leaders? Naomi Oreskes and Erik M. Conway attempted to do this in their book *Merchants of Doubt*, which discusses the shameful behavior of scientists in defending the tobacco industry and disputing the reality of climate change. They point out that although scientists, sometimes with impressive credentials like Duesberg and Séralini, are often the charismatic leaders misleading us, they generally have not done any scientific work in the area in which they are declaiming. With respect to scientists who tried to convince us that cigarette smoking is not harmful, they note,

Over the course of more than twenty years, these men did almost no original scientific research on any of the issues on which they weighed in. Once they had been prominent researchers, but by the time they turned to the topics of our story, they were mostly attacking the work and the reputations of others.[60]

In fact, many of these scientists seem to have fallen off the rails. Although Séralini did publish a study on a GMO product, his credentials were never in this kind of toxicology and in fact he apparently did almost everything possible incorrectly. Duesberg was past his most productive scientific days when he began railing against HIV as the cause of AIDS and was trained in chemistry, not virology or medicine. Wakefield, a gastroenterologist, should never have been given credence as a knowledgeable source regarding a disorder that involves the central nervous system like autism. Neither LaPierre nor McCarthy has any scientific credentials. This pattern will not always work, but in the case of these five leaders, their opinions are not actually "expert," despite their credentials in loosely related fields.

Another tactic of these charismatic leaders is to vociferously accuse the rest of the scientific community of bullying them. Again, Oreskes and Conway give the example of Frederick Seitz, the scientist hired by the tobacco industry who spent years trying to convince regulatory authorities and the public that smoking and lung cancer are unrelated. Seitz of course was roundly criticized and ostracized by mainstream scientists as the connection became all too clear. "Seitz justified his increasing social and intellectual isolation by blaming others. American science had become 'rigid,' he insisted, his colleagues dogmatic and close-minded."[61]

As we have seen in LaPierre's case, charismatic leaders actually distract us from the core issues by avoiding the messiness of data analysis and broadening their rhetoric to universal concerns about freedom and justice. They try to scare us, telling us that we are, like them, sorry victims of dastardly forces, and they lay out for us the enemy we can unite against: big companies, liberals, other scientists, and the mentally ill. Against them, all science has are rigorously designed and conducted experiments, data analyses with equations that can fill a page, and the seemingly endless presentation of new facts. It doesn't seem like a fair fight.

I Know You're Wrong, but I'm Going to Copy You Anyway

No discussion of the charismatic leader would be complete without considering the psychology of the group that forms around him or her. As we discussed earlier in this chapter, many theories of leadership focus on the ways in which followers' perception of a leader determine his or her actual authority. Once we think about the intensive ways in which the charismatic leader formulates an "us" as opposed to a "them," we must then examine what happens to people's decision making and rational thinking capacities when they join groups.

When discussing groups, it is essential to recognize that, as Gestalt theorists have argued, the group is more than the sum of its parts. Groups have *higher-order emergent properties*, which are characteristics that can be observed *only* when the group comes together and not when considering the members of a group individually. Group focus on a particular task or on the message of a speaker is a good example of an emergent property. Engagement on the individual level is not the same as the engagement of the group as a whole. This kind of emergent property is something that defines the group as different from the aggregation of its individual members.[62]

But how do individuals join groups, and what psychological process occurs as they identify increasingly with the group? Many social psychologists have noted that the simple act of individuals categorizing themselves as group members is enough to cause group behavior and all of the psychological processes that accompany group formation.[63] This means that it is relatively easy for a group to form—in fact, it represents one of our most natural inclinations as humans. In today's world, triggers for group psychology are particularly abundant, considering how easy it is to join a "group" with a click of a button on Facebook, LinkedIn, Twitter, and many other forms of social media. The ability to join a "Green Our Vaccines" or "No GMOs" group on Facebook reduces some of the barriers that may exist in traditional group formation, such as geographic location and time commitments. If psychologists are correct that this simple act of self-categorization as a group member is enough to produce group behavior and group psychology, then we can begin to realize how important it is to conceive of some of these health denialist movements as "group" activities and the appropriateness of applying principles of group psychology to them.

The first step in the process of becoming identified as a group member has often been called "depersonalization." The self comes to be seen in terms of membership in a group. This process leads people to behave in terms of a self-image as a psychological representative of a group rather than as an individual.[64] Joining the group is an extremely adaptive human behavior. It allows us to make sense of a lot of worldly phenomena that might be complex or confusing. In particular, group membership allows for *social reality testing*, in which we can move from an opinion such as "I think global warming is a serious problem" to an affirmation that "Global warming is a serious problem" by looking to the opinions of our fellow group members as a test of the idea.[65] To some extent, we suspend the imperative to dive deeply into an issue in order to form an opinion when we join a group because we assume that the group has already done this. The more impressive sounding the group's name, the more persuasive is this assumption. "National Rifle Association" sounds more official than "Gun Owner's Club," for example.

It seems logical that a person's identification with a group will be shaken when groups with countervailing views crop up, but this is not generally the case. Group identities paradoxically become stronger as people encounter those that seem opposite or somehow very different from themselves. For example, in one study, two researchers organized people into either same-sex pairs (male-male or female-female) or four-person groups (two males and two females). Subjects were more likely to define themselves in gender-based terms in the four-person group than in the same-sex pairs. Once women were confronted with men, they began to identify more precisely as women than when they were simply paired with another woman.[66] An anti-vaccine group will become more strongly identified as anti-vaccine when faced with a pro-vaccine group, even if the latter offers evidence to support its opinions. This is a basic tenet of group psychology. As such, when charismatic leaders try to emphasize the presence of the opposition and even try to engage with them, they are effectively stimulating patterns of group psychology that will strengthen group identity in the presence of a group perceived as very different.

Once a group identity is formed, people tend to want to conform to the group's opinions, even when those opinions are obviously wrong. A few classic experiments have demonstrated the power of the conformity effect. In one early experiment, Muzafer Sherif used the autokinetic effect to demonstrate how group conformity can influence individual perceptions and behavior. The autokinetic effect is an optical illusion in which pinpoints of light seem to move when projected in a dark room. Generally, every individual will have a different perception of how much the light moved, and these perceptions can really be quite distinct. Sherif found very distinctive perceptions of how far the light moved among his subjects until he brought them together and tried the experiment again. Once they were brought together, subjects' reports on how far the light moved converged on an agreement point somewhere in the middle of all of their differing perceptions.[67] This experiment does not make clear whether people's perceptions actually change or whether they simply report what they think will be most conforming and most socially acceptable to the group. However, many years after Sherif's experiments, neuroscientists continue to demonstrate that individual cognitive perceptions can actually be altered in the presence of group conformity pressures.

Gregory S. Berns and colleagues at Emory University have shown that when people change their minds about something to conform to peer pressure, even when the change means adopting false beliefs, the parts of the brain involved in perception—the occipital-parietal network—are activated.[68] On the other hand, activity in the decision-making part of the brain—the PFC—is actually suppressed when this switch occurs. This means that when we bow to social pressure there is an actual change in perception—how we see the facts—rather than a reasoned decision to change our minds.

Solomon Asch characterized a more dramatic example of social conformity in the 1950s. A single subject was seated around a table with a group of experiment confederates. Everyone was shown one piece of paper with a line on it and then another piece of paper with three lines on it. The task was to identify which line on the second piece of paper was the same length as that on the first piece of paper. Participants went around the table and gave their responses. Seating was arranged so that the subject always answered last, after all of the confederates. The confederates and subject gave the correct answer for a number of trials. After a certain number of trials, however, the confederates would begin to give a blatantly incorrect response.

Asch found that 75% of naïve subjects gave an incorrect answer to at least one question when preceded by the incorrect answers of confederates. When interviewing the experimental subjects after the experiment, Asch found different categories of "yielders" (those who answered incorrectly after hearing the incorrect responses of confederates). Some participants reacted with *distortion of perception*. These participants believed that the incorrect responses were actually true. These subjects represented a very small proportion of the yielders. Others displayed a *distortion of judgment*, in which they became convinced that the majority must be right and then changed their answers, mostly due to low confidence and extreme doubt. The third group displayed a *distortion of action*, suggesting that they knew the correct answer but answered incorrectly in order to conform to the group. Asch's experiment was instrumental in showing the strong, almost universal, drive to conform, even when we realize that the majority view is incorrect.

Hey There, Sports Fans

As we discuss throughout the book, these kinds of irrational or incorrect perceptions can, in certain instances, serve a societal purpose. They often allow us to function in social units and to form groups that offer protection, relief from stress, monetary benefits, and a whole host of other survival advantages. A simple example is found among fans of a particular sports team. Members of such groups believe that their team *deserves* to win the championship on the basis of some divine right. They buy jerseys, T-shirts, and hats with the team logo and insist that their team is the best. There may be no evidence that their team is indeed superior to others, nor is there any reason to assume that supernatural forces take sides in these things, so sports team affiliations might be characterized as largely irrational. And yet, these affiliations serve to bind together people who might otherwise have nothing in common, offering them the opportunity to relate to a large and otherwise diverse group. For many people, the experience is quite fulfilling and it certainly generates a great deal of income for the team's owner(s).

In short, conforming to the group, even if that means distorting reality, may serve a highly adaptive purpose. It is part of a human inclination that allows people to set aside their differences, come together, and form units that serve as the foundation of functioning human societies. Forming these units comes naturally to us, and we may benefit from them in ways that enhance our survival, including gaining monetary support for families, forming militaries to fight off enemies, and generally creating a social infrastructure that allows people to come to our aid when we collapse in the street. The problem is that we may find it difficult to turn off this urge to conform in situations in which it is not appropriate. In particular, the urge to conform becomes particularly dangerous when we are trying to sort out complex evidence on a scientific issue. In this situation, conformity and group formation does not function in a productive manner but rather has the capacity to distract from and distort reality. Until there is a group whose sole rationale is to seriously and objectively evaluate the scientific merit of health claims and come to evidence-based conclusions that are flexible in the face of new data, group membership generally does little to advance our understanding of what science tells us. This is potentially remediable. Why not start groups—from small community associations to national organizations—whose main function is to help people feel warm, involved, and accepted in the joint exploration of science as it affects our decision making? When the claim is made, for example, that eating gluten-free food is better for all of us (and not just for people suffering with celiac disease), joining a "science exploration" group would function to allow people to work together to figure out what the evidence shows. The group could bring in experts, read articles in popular but respected journals like *Scientific American*, and figure out together if there is anything to it. When that task is done, the group could move onto another issue, say, whether global warming is real.

In addition to the practical benefits that group membership provides us, there are profound psychological benefits, particularly the availability of comfort. Human personalities come in every imaginable variety, of course, but in general we are a social and gregarious species that shuns isolation. Whenever we experience fear, worry, and pain, it is our instinct to seek comfort from others. As Brian G. Southwell puts it, "Much of the discussion we seek with others in moments of elevated emotion . . . is not necessarily focused on new factual information sharing as much as it is focused on reassurance, coping with stress, and ritualistic bonding."[69]

After a charismatic leader like Wayne LaPierre terrifies us with images of armed hooligans lurking around every corner, he then offers us the comfort of joining his organization, the NRA, and finding safety with others in similar danger. Neuroscientists have established that social affiliations in mammals, including humans, involve the hormone oxytocin, sometimes referred to as the "love hormone."[70] Forming group affiliations stimulates the release of oxytocin in the brain, which, as Ernst Fehr of the University of Zurich and Colin Camerer of the California Institute of Technology point out, "seems to limit the fear of betrayal in social interactions."[71] They speculate, based on animal studies, that oxytocin may reduce amygdala activity in order to reduce the fear of betrayal. Thus, the same hormone that is critical in all mammalian species for pair-bonding and maternal behavior may also work to make people feel "loved" when they are in a group, regardless of whether that group is feeding them misleading information or promoting scientific thinking.

Group membership can change the way you think by two processes: informational influence and normative influence. Both are probably at play in most instances of health science denialism. Informational influence indicates a desire to conform to the group because you think the group may be correct about something. This form of influence is strong when people are uncertain about what is correct and incorrect, generally takes place in private, and is particularly strong with the first few members of the group you encounter.[72] For example, if you are not sure whether GMOs cause cancer, you would be particularly prone to this type of influence. The first person from an anti-GMO group you meet would have the most influence on your opinions, and by the time you met the 20th person in the group, you would be hearing the same opinions repeated that you are already convinced are true. Informational influence is therefore especially strong upon first encounter with an individual who has an opinion. The mother who is uncertain about whether vaccines are safe for her child is particularly prone to being persuaded that they are not if she suddenly encounters even a single member of an anti-vaccine group. This is why demographics are important in patterns of health beliefs. If you are uncertain about the truth of a medical claim and you are likely to meet someone with a strong anti-establishment opinion because of where you live, then you yourself are also more likely to take on this view as soon as you meet someone who harbors it. Irrational denial of medical fact is thus particularly spurred on by informational influence, since the complicated nature of scientific discovery makes it more likely that people will be uncertain about what is in fact correct.

Normative influence has to do with wanting to be accepted in a group. This kind of influence is what most clearly explains Sherif's findings. Even if you know that members of the group are blatantly incorrect, you will actively agree with them in order to maintain an acceptable social status. This kind of influence is normally observed as groups become larger and mainly influences behavior that takes place in front of the entire group rather than in private.[73] In other words, you may privately believe that the group is incorrect about something but you will nevertheless publicly proclaim that it is in fact correct.[74] As the group grows, you are more likely to feel a stronger need to be accepted. There is probably an element of this type of influence in many health science denialist groups as well, whether or not people realize it consciously. Some members of health science denialist groups may feel that the group's assumptions are incorrect but maintain a position of advocacy of the group's stance in order to avoid being excluded. This kind of influence is especially potent within social networks: if all the mothers on your block believe that vaccines cause autism and hold a rally against vaccines, you are more likely to join them, even if on some level you believe that the premise of their argument could be flawed. Pair this instinct with the fact that the science behind vaccination is incredibly complex and you are more likely to be influenced by this group on a basic informational level as well.

There are a number of theories about why we are so ready to conform to the group, even in situations in which its views are clearly wrong. In the case of followers of charismatic leaders, great uncertainty and psychological distress are key factors that make people prone to these leaders' influence. In fact, some leadership theorists have hypothesized that charismatic leadership cannot even exist in the absence of a crisis.[75] The novelty of a charismatic leader's message as well as the uncertainty felt by the listener will often have a strong effect on how well the listener receives the message and how convincing it seems.[76] Uncertainty is most definitely a feature of health science denialism. Unsure about what causes cancer or autism, we may feel comforted in believing a strong leader's message that GMOs or vaccines, respectively, are the answer. In the case of anti-vaccine sentiment, parents whose children suffer from autism, epilepsy, or other disorders now frequently attributed by these groups to vaccines are clearly under conditions of high stress and psychological pain. The uncertainty surrounding the complexities of science as well as the mysteries of complex, chronic diseases and the psychological distress surrounding their management all create a perfect environment for the dissemination of strong anti-establishment messages from a charismatic leader. These conditions also create a ripe environment for high levels of social conformity of the sort Asch observed.

A Shot Against Persuasion

What should we do when faced with the persuasive tactics of a highly charismatic leader? Is it possible to resist persuasion? Although there has been far more research on being persuaded than on resisting persuasion, psychologists have found that it is possible to avoid persuasion.[77] Resistance to persuasion has been described in the same terms as resistance to certain illnesses after vaccination. A person can be inoculated against persuasion by fabricating counterarguments, being forewarned about an upcoming persuasive message, and simply taking time to think alone after hearing a persuasive message before taking any action. In particular, just as a person is inoculated against a virus by receiving weakened doses of the virus itself and then mounting an immune response against it, we can be inoculated against persuasive arguments by being exposed to weaker versions of those arguments and then being encouraged to generate counterarguments.[78]

One group of theorists has identified what they call the "persuasion knowledge model." The persuasion knowledge model refers to the ways in which people process powerful messages and recognize the sources and processes of persuasion occurring. The theory suggests that people learn "coping" techniques to deal with persuasive messages that can be cultivated and change over time. Coping techniques may help individuals separate emotion from their evaluation of the message, refocus their attention on a part of the message that seems more significant to them rather than what the persuader is trying to emphasize, elucidate the chain of events that led to the persuasive message, or make judgments about the persuader's goals and tactics.[79]

Other experiments have suggested that the cognitive resources of an individual have a major influence on whether or not he or she is persuaded by a message. *Cognitive load* refers to the amount of strain on someone's cognitive resources. In experiments, someone who is forced to memorize a very long string of numbers would be in the high cognitive load condition, and someone who is forced to memorize a very short string of numbers would be in the low cognitive load condition. The point of these manipulations is to see how the effects of persuasion alter when people are more or less distracted. One study tried to assess the ability of subjects to resist persuasion depending on the extent of their cognitive loads. In one condition, subjects were told about a new drug called *AspirinForte*, which had received bad press due to its unpleasant taste and its damaging effects on the environment when produced in mass quantities. These subjects were then told to memorize a long string of numbers (the high cognitive load condition) and next were exposed to an ad for *AspirinForte* and told to write down as many arguments against the use of the product as possible. In the other condition, subjects were asked to memorize a short string of letters (the low cognitive load condition) and then were exposed to the ad and asked to come up with arguments against the drug. The experimenters then collected data on the certainty of subjects in their attitudes toward the drug. They found that people with a high cognitive load were less certain about their attitudes toward the drug, even if they rated the source of the advertisement as highly trustworthy. In addition, those in the low cognitive load condition had higher-quality counterarguments, as judged on persuasiveness by external analysts, even though those in the high cognitive load condition had a greater absolute number of counterarguments.[80] This all suggests that difficulties with resisting persuasion are related to factors other than the source of the argument. The condition of people receiving the message, how knowledgeable they are about the topic, and how distracted they are will all affect their ability to think about counterarguments that might prevent them from being completely persuaded. Perhaps counterintuitively, the more tired, stressed out, and busy you are, the more likely you are to be convinced by persuasive messages simply because you do not have the energy to come up with better ones of your own.

There is some evidence that making people aware of the way in which they are processing persuasive messages and the biases with which they are engaging can help them rethink their attitudes. In one experiment, researchers exposed subjects to a message from either a likeable or dislikeable source. Some subjects were specifically told not to let "non-message" factors affect their judgment of the message. When subjects were already being persuaded by a peripheral route that depended on non-message perceptions such as the authority of the speaker, being alerted to the possible existence of bias resulted in more careful scrutiny of the message and less bias in interpreting it.[81]

The results of these types of experiments suggest that there is room to intervene in the process of persuasion. Several possibilities for encouraging more careful scrutiny of the particularly persuasive messages of charismatic leaders exist. For example, nurses and doctors dealing with parents who are afraid of vaccinating their children might try attitude inoculation. Rather than simply arguing with the parent, the healthcare provider might offer weakened versions of arguments the parent may have heard against vaccines. The doctor or nurse might even be trained to present these views in a highly noncharismatic, flat manner. Research shows that when inundated with weakened versions of a persuasive argument, people are able to mount effective counterarguments against them. The healthcare provider would then encourage the parent to come back at a later date to discuss the possibility of vaccination again. In the interim, when the parent is faced with anti-vaccine messages, he or she will be more likely to mount effective counterarguments against them and more likely to return to the doctor with a changed attitude. This strategy would of course not work with everyone. People who are already entrenched in anti-vaccine attitudes or face significant social pressure not to vaccinate their children might not be swayed by this strategy. However, such a strategy would likely work for the parents who are simply unsure and are at risk of being persuaded by anti-vaccine activists. These types of parents represent a larger and more vulnerable group than the group of people who are already firmly convinced of the danger of vaccines. If we could get the parents on the fence to decide to vaccinate their children, we could probably avert many of the frightening gaps in vaccine coverage we are seeing today.

This type of "inoculation" might proceed as follows:

PARENT : I have heard that vaccines can cause serious brain damage in children, like autism, and I am not sure that I want my child to be vaccinated.

NURSE : Yes, there are definitely some people out there who have claimed that vaccines cause autism. Their evidence for this is that there has been an increase in autism over the last few years; that vaccines used to have a small amount of a mercury preservative and large, repeated doses of mercury can harm the brain; and that there are some parents who insist that their children started showing signs of autism after receiving a vaccine. Now that you have heard these arguments, you might want to do a little research and see what the evidence is for them. I would be happy to help you with this and to talk with you again about your concerns. Why don't we make an appointment to discuss your thoughts and concerns soon?

For individuals who are faced with confusing, conflicting scientific messages, we recommend a few strategies. Take a moment, step back, and think about how you are processing the information in front of you. Do you have Jenny McCarthy on the TV in the background while you clean your house, talk on the phone, and make dinner for your children? Or have you sat down, listened to the arguments with a clear head, and given yourself ample time to think about possible counterarguments? Is it possible that you are exercising any biases? When making an important decision about your health and wellness, such as whether or not to buy a gun or to allow your family member to be treated with ECT, it might be wise to take a moment to list any possible biases you might have when receiving information about these topics. Who told you that ECT caused brain damage? Could they have any possible biases? What non-message factors might have influenced your perception of their message? This kind of simple reflective thinking can go a long way in helping to make sure you are not simply persuaded by charisma and bias but that you have truly thought through the facts and have remained aware of all of your potential cognitive pitfalls along the way. It is also important to identify sources of stress, both related to the health issue at hand or in general, to which you are being subjected. Reasonable decisions, as we have shown above, are best made when cognitive load is minimized.

Noreena Hertz, in her very useful book *Eyes Wide Open*, discusses how encouraging people to calmly consider alternative points of view can have a very powerful effect:

> Studies show that simply by posing such "imagine if" questions, which allow us to consider alternative explanations and different perspectives, we can distance ourselves from the frames, cues, anchors and rhetoric that might be affecting us. Liberated from these tricks and triggers, we can consider information through a more neutral, less emotive, more analytical and nuanced lens.[82]

From the point of view of public health measures, it is critical that any attempt to limit the influence of charismatic leaders take into considerable account the powerful effect those leaders have in making us feel safe, understood, and even loved. We have indicated that the more fear a charismatic leader is able to conjure in a potential acolyte, the more powerful is the activation of select brain circuits that will make it difficult for countervailing evidence to have an impact. Charismatic leaders induce brain changes that first heighten the fear centers of the brain, like the amygdala, and then suppress the decision-making areas in the PFC. Those brain changes also contribute to an increased release of oxytocin that gives us a feeling of belonging and comfort. Dry, pedantic harangues about data will be powerless in the face of these potent effects. Rather, it is critical to make people feel that by using their minds to evaluate scientific claims they are joining a welcoming club of people who trust the scientific method and attempt to get at the truth about what is healthy.

Resisting persuasion requires a kind of self-awareness and critical thinking that is not necessarily intuitive or natural. But learning how to think critically in this way can help anyone in any career or walk of life, not just in resisting anti-science viewpoints. Therefore, it would make sense if middle school and high school curricula included more time developing these skills. As we advocate throughout this book, rather than focusing so heavily on memorization, schools should teach children the techniques to think through complex problems. Children should learn how to identify a flawed experimental design or a flawed argument, to become aware of how they process arguments, and to formulate viable counterarguments and test ideas. Spending more time on debate techniques, requiring children to argue against something they may intuitively believe, or even simply teaching children about rhetoric and the psychology behind persuasion would all aid in developing useful critical thinking skills. Cultivating critical thinking and awareness of cognitive traps and biases not only helps us identify faulty scientific arguments but also helps us to become better decision makers, better thinkers, and better-informed citizens.

Confirmation Bias

O NE OF AMERICA'S GREATEST SCIENTISTS SUMMARIZED
confirmation bias well when he quipped, "I wouldn't have seen
it if I didn't believe it."

That scientist was the great Hall of Famer and New York Yankee
baseball player Yogi Berra. How do we know Yogi Berra said that?
One of us once heard someone say that he did, and it sounds like the
kind of thing that has been attributed to him. Of course, there are
those who say that Yogi didn't say many of the things attributed
to him and that there are actually perfectly logical explanations
for some of the seemingly nonsensical statements he allegedly
did utter.[1] But we don't care about any of that. We love the line, it
makes our point well, and we are going to stick to the Yogi attribu-
tion no matter what kind of disconfirming evidence crops up. As
Yogi might have said, "When you come to a piece of evidence that
doesn't agree with what you already believe, tear it to shreds and
then ignore it."

Confirmation bias refers to our tendency to attend only to information that agrees with what we already think is true. Notice that
we did not simply say that this bias involves ignoring evidence that
is incompatible with our beliefs but rather that it is an active process
in which we selectively pay attention to those things that confirm

our hypotheses. Confirmation bias is responsible for not only a great deal of denial of scientific evidence but also the actual generation and maintenance of incorrect scientific information. That is, scientists, doctors, and public health experts are as prone as anyone else is to "seeing what we believe," making it especially difficult to help people sort out what is true science from the mistakes and outright fabrications. As we will see, confirmation bias is strongly rooted in primitive needs and emotion and therefore not amenable to correction merely by reciting facts.

Although confirmation bias is irrational in the sense that it does not take into consideration evidence, it is still frequently adaptive and even necessary. Sometimes rejecting something because of an initial bad impression when there is an alternative that suits our needs well is time-saving, even if the reasons behind our rejection are not evidence-based. If we got gastrointestinal symptoms once after eating a particular brand of canned baked beans, there is no harm in automatically picking a different brand the next time, even if more careful consideration would reveal that the original brand was not responsible for making us sick. Confirmation bias is one of those cognitive techniques that enable us to make rapid decisions. In everyday life that can be an advantage; when making decisions about scientific truth, however, it rarely is. Specific networks in the human brain reinforce positions we take because of confirmation bias, networks that have evolved to keep us safe and happy. Challenging these ideas requires substantial mental effort and energy expenditure that we cannot be expected to sustain on a regular basis.

The everyday, practical use of confirmation bias to make necessary decisions runs counter to something at the very heart of the scientific method: disconfirmation. Science operates mostly by creating hypotheses based on what is already known and then generating data in an attempt to prove the hypothesis is wrong. Only after exhaustive attempts to disconfirm the hypothesis have failed do scientists begin to think it might be correct. Although as we shall see that confirmation bias is used by scientists—sometimes generating incorrect inferences—the very nature of science resists acceptance of anything just because it is what is already believed. Proper science is a long, exhausting, and often frustrating process in which experiments fail over and over again. In other words, science is a continuous process of trying one's best to prove that everything we believe is wrong. Only when repeated rigorous attempts to do so prove fruitless do we begin to believe a scientific theory might just be true.

In this chapter we will demonstrate how confirmation bias, although a highly adaptive human trait, actually often causes scientific misperceptions due to our resistance to the often counterintuitive disconfirmation process of scientific inquiry. The chapter explains confirmation bias and why it is adaptive as a form of learning from experience. We then explore the ways in which confirmation bias affects health beliefs with a particular focus on scientific and medical professionals who are by no means immune to its power. We follow this by exploring some reasons, both social and biological, why confirmation bias exists. Finally, we propose some ways of countering confirmation bias.

What Is Confirmation Bias?

Confirmation bias crops up in everyone's life on a regular basis. Let us say, for example, that we have decided that a person we recently met, we will call him Sherlock, is very smart. We came to this conclusion because at a party he corrected someone who claimed that global warming is just the natural result of the end of the last ice age and therefore nothing to worry about. Sherlock calmly and clearly explained that the last ice age ended about 10,000 years ago and that all mathematical analyses have shown that although the earth warmed up after it was over, this does not account for the global warming we are experiencing today. Hence, Sherlock soberly and dispassionately concluded, we have a lot to worry about.

Sherlock sounded very confident in what he said. He spoke clearly. Furthermore, he has a deep voice and is taller than average. There was something "authoritative" about him. And of course, his name contributed to an overall sense that Sherlock is indeed a very smart person.

We subsequently see Sherlock several times at parties and meetings. Every time he speaks, we pay close attention to what he says, agreeing with every point he makes. During one such gathering, Sherlock explains that pasteurization destroys the vitamin D that milk naturally contains. He says this is so because vitamin D is a fat-soluble vitamin.

"Think of what happens when you broil a steak," he tells us, as we sit raptly listening to him. "The fat melts and is discarded. That is what happens to the vitamin D when they heat it up to temperatures like you have in your oven."

This seems correct, especially because we remember learning that vitamin D is indeed a fat- as opposed to a water-soluble vitamin like vitamin C. The next day, however, someone who was also at the party mentions to us that Sherlock was wrong.

"First of all," Martha tells us, "milk does not have vitamin D in it until the manufacturers add it in. They have been doing that since the 1930s. Second of all, pasteurization doesn't involve temperatures anywhere near what you get in your oven. Pasteurized milk is not heated beyond the boiling point because it would curdle. The usual method of pasteurization involves heating the milk to 72°C for 15 seconds. Finally, pasteurization doesn't lower vitamin D levels by any amount that makes a difference."

Now, Martha does not have a deep and alluring voice like Sherlock, and she is not as tall as he is. Furthermore, as we are listening to her we are trying to rush out to an important business meeting. Martha's speech is full of details, and we simply do not have the attention right now for them. Who cares how long they have been pasteurizing milk, and how much is 72°C converted to Fahrenheit degrees? We notice that she says "any amount that makes a difference," and we immediately think, "So it does lower the vitamin D content by *some* amount." Sherlock was right—Martha even admitted it.

As we drive to our next meeting, our blood begins to boil. Martha is always attacking people, always trying to find the worst she can in them. She is probably envious of Sherlock because he is smarter and more popular. Every time thereafter when someone tries to disagree with something Sherlock says, we feel that same rush of angry emotion as we did in the car contemplating Martha's attack on him and we barely consider the contradictory information. Our belief that Sherlock is smart is repeatedly confirmed and becomes unshakeable.

This example of confirmation bias illustrates several of its properties. First, it is prone to the *irrational primacy effect*: we give more credence to what we hear or experience first than everything that follows. As Raymond S. Nickerson puts it, "When a person must draw a conclusion on the basis of information acquired and integrated over time, the information acquired early in the process is likely to carry more weight than that acquired later."[2] Our first experience with Sherlock was a positive one in which he was in fact correct. Global warming today cannot be attributed to any lingering effects of the ending of the last ice age. Second, confirmation bias is subject to emotion. We were incidentally experiencing positive emotions when we first met Sherlock. We were at a party, and we were relaxed and having fun. Sherlock is tall, handsome, and well-spoken. By contrast, we were harried when we spoke to Martha, whom we experience with negative emotion. Third, in order to maintain our conviction that Sherlock is smart, we fail to listen to anything that contradicts this judgment. Instead, we summon up our angry defense of him. As it turns out, Sherlock is completely wrong on the pasteurization issue. Perhaps Martha did not need to add all those details, which only increased our sense that she is a pedantic irritant. But even though we do not yet know the facts—we have done no independent research of our own—we instinctively believe Sherlock and not Martha.

It turns out that Sherlock had just read something about global warming in a magazine in his dentist's office before coming to the party. Otherwise, he knows very little about science and frequently insists on assumptions that are untrue. But the more we are confronted with that fact, the more it would be embarrassing to have to admit that we have been wrong about him. If we acknowledge that we were wrong about Sherlock and that despite his name he is really a blowhard, then perhaps everyone will be mad at us for defending him and we will look stupid. So we cling to our defense of Sherlock, becoming more and more polarized in our view that he is smart and that everyone else is misjudging him. And thus is revealed another, very serious effect of the confirmation bias: it polarizes people. Ideally, whenever someone asserts a "fact" about an unfamiliar topic, we should maintain a healthy skepticism, ask questions, and even look into it further on our own so that we can come to our own conclusions. When scientists do this together to get an answer to a question it is called collaboration. Confirmation bias, on the other hand, is an anti-collaboration phenomenon. Each person or group of people stridently defends its own position, thus increasingly driving everyone further apart.

If you think back, you will almost certainly identify times in your life when you have been prone to confirmation bias. Maybe it happened when you judged a person or decided to buy something. Perhaps you set your sights on renting a particular apartment because you loved the big windows in the living room that let sunlight in on a beautiful summer afternoon. After that, you rationalized the fact that the rent was a bit high by noting that it was only a bit higher than a friend's new apartment; you dismissed what looked like a water stain on the ceiling in the bedroom by assuming it happened a long time ago during a rare terrible storm; and you overlooked a cockroach scurrying across the living room floor. All of this was set aside because your very first visit to the apartment was emotionally favorable. It did not even occur to you that all that sunlight would stream through only on sunny afternoons when you are usually at work. Fortunately, someone else got the apartment before you could put down a deposit, and that poor soul is now fighting with the landlord to fix the leak in the upstairs apartment that is dripping into the ceiling of the bedroom and to get an exterminator in to fight the vermin infestation. Perhaps that unfortunate renter would have benefited from some wisdom articulated more than 700 years ago by Dante. In the *Divine Comedy*, St. Thomas Aquinas cautions Dante when they meet in Paradise, "Opinion—hasty—often can incline to the wrong side, and then affection for one's own opinion binds, confines the mind."[3]

Confirmation bias can and does also affect how we think about our health. In a study published in the *Proceedings of the National Academy of Medicine* researchers followed patients for more than a year and found there was absolutely no relationship between their arthritis pain and the weather.[4] We doubt that the publication of this paper 20 years ago has influenced any patient or her doctor to abandon the notion that inclement weather makes joints ache more. That belief was probably embedded in people's minds hundreds of years ago—everyone has no doubt heard it articulated by his or her grandparents. Once this idea is implanted in our minds, we ignore every bit of evidence that contradicts it, even though there really is no biological basis for such an assertion. Once we understand what is actually involved in the two main forms of arthritis, osteoarthritis (in which joints degenerate with age) and rheumatoid arthritis (an autoimmune disease caused by abnormal antibodies attacking joints that can begin at any age), it becomes very hard to understand how humidity, cloudiness, or precipitation could possibly be a factor in the progression of the disease. Yet we are fully capable of falsely associating bad weather with pain because that is what we already think is the case. Fortunately, not much harm is done by believing this, although if arthritis sufferers take too much medication or avoid recommended therapy and exercise just because the weather is bad, there could be consequences.

As we noted earlier, confirmation bias is not without advantages, which is perhaps why it remains a part of the human panoply of cognitive devices. We need to use our experience, the things we have learned in the past and know in the present, to guide us in almost everything we do. If we bought a product that turns out to have been defective, we are biased against purchasing that product again. That is, every time we see that product in the store—let's say it is an expensive umbrella that allegedly withstands 30-mile-an-hour winds but in fact collapsed the first time it was exposed to a slight breeze—we immediately notice its flaws and this ensures that we don't make the same mistake twice.[5] Of course, it is entirely possible that the umbrella we bought was the only defective one the manufacturer made. Hence, our decision not to buy this umbrella based on previous experience is technically biased. Without evaluating a large number of this manufacturer's umbrellas we cannot really be sure if there are any good ones or not. But no one would fault us for relying on confirmation bias in this instance. Who wants to take a chance on getting deceived again when there are so many alternative products (like a cheap umbrella that will handle at least a 2-mile-per-hour wind)? It is easy to think of many instances, from trivial to those of great importance in our lives, in which confirmation bias enables us to use experience to make quick and adaptive decisions.

So we all are prone to confirmation bias, but in this chapter we want to reinforce our point that intelligence is not a factor in the penchant to deny scientific evidence. So we use two examples that involve people who are generally believed to be smart and even have special training in the fields involved: physicians' overprescribing of antibiotics and health scientists' tenacious insistence that eating fat is the cause of heart disease.

Confirmation Bias Among Scientists

Science, too, operates in large measure by relying on experience. When a scientist (or more likely today a team of scientists) completes an experiment or analyzes existing data in a new way, something will emerge. Most of the time what emerges is of little interest— more experiments fail than succeed, which is why scientists labor so long on the same thing and why graduate students in science suffer so much, hoping that one of their experiments will rise to sufficient significance to finally merit a dissertation that gets them their PhDs. But if the results are interesting, the scientists will write up their findings in a scientific paper and submit the paper to a scientific journal. The editor of the journal will look it over and decide whether the paper has a chance of being published in the journal and, if it does, will send it to several independent experts in the field for peer review. These experts are usually called *referees* and journals that use this system are known as *refereed journals*. Most papers come back from review with recommendations that they be rejected. The most prestigious scientific journals in the health field reject between 80% and 90% of the papers they receive. Hence, it is a tough road from writing a paper to getting it published.

A paper that does get published, however, may be read widely by other scientists. The new findings now have some authority by virtue of being published, and the more prestigious the journal the more they will be noticed and seen as important.[6] It will now become imperative that other scientists in the field take these findings into account when they do their own work. If another group performs an experiment whose findings agree with the published ones, this is called a *replication*. If the new results are not confirmatory, however, it is said that the second group of investigators has *failed to replicate* the original findings and it is incumbent upon them to explain why they got a different result. Notice that there is already a bit of a bias in the way this works—even if the follow-up experiment was done with nearly perfect scientific rigor, the word *failure* is used if it yields a different result than a previously published one. There is, then, the opportunity for confirmation bias because no one wants to be a "failure," even though in fact a well-executed experiment that yields a discrepant finding can hardly be called a "failure." It is really just different.

The use of confirmation bias has its advantages in science, as it does in daily life. Using previously published findings to guide future experiments narrows the field of exploration and increases the chances of finding something. It is very rare nowadays that anyone stumbles on a finding by accident, the way Edward Jenner did in the late 18th century when he discovered the smallpox vaccine. Rather, today's science works by building upon previous findings until something of value develops. The scientists who developed the vaccine for the human papillomavirus (HPV), for example, knew from previous work HPV's role in the development of cervical cancer, its molecular structure, and the way in which immune cells attack viruses. They were then able to use this information to design a method of extracting just the viral proteins necessary to cause the body to manufacture neutralizing antibodies without being capable of causing actual infection. In other words, these investigators were guided in what to look for each step of the way by what had been published in the past. When they stumbled upon a discrepant finding, their first assumption would have been to wonder if they did something wrong in performing the experiment and figure out how to fix it, not to trash the whole idea. To do otherwise would have been to throw unnecessary obstacles into the process. Thus, scientists use confirmation bias in order to benefit from previous findings in pushing ahead with a discovery process.

But of course, just as is the case in daily life, confirmation bias can have negative consequences for both science and medicine. Sometimes, a finding or hypothesis gets so enshrined by scientists that they resist accepting evidence that proves it incorrect. Doctors can become so convinced of a belief that actual evidence does not dissuade them and they continue a practice that is not only useless but even harmful. "People sometimes see in data the patterns for which they are looking, regardless of whether the patterns are really there," wrote Raymond S. Nickerson of Tufts University, an expert on confirmation bias.[7] One example is the administration of antibiotics.

Confirmation Bias in the Medical Field: Antibiotic Overuse

The famous discovery by Alexander Fleming in 1928 that the *Penicillium* mold inhibited the growth of bacteria in a petri dish was not in fact as "out of the blue" as is often believed. The term *antibiosis* was coined in the 19th century when biologists noticed that bacteria produce substances that inhibit other bacteria. That various fungi inhibited the growth of bacteria had also been reported before Fleming made his breakthrough finding. Penicillin was not even the first antibiotic introduced. Sulfonamides were introduced in 1932, with penicillin not becoming available to civilians until after World War II. There is no question, however, that antibiotics are the closest thing to "miracle" drugs ever invented. They have changed the face of human interaction with bacteria that cause infection, saving countless lives since the middle of the 20th century and causing relatively minor and infrequent complications or adverse side effects.

Since 1950, then, we have lived in an era blessed with a class of medications that have turned previously serious and sometimes fatal diseases like bacterial pneumonia, strep throat,[8] and syphilis into curable illness. Furthermore, antibiotics rarely seemed to harm anyone. There is the occasional person who is allergic to penicillin or other antibiotics, and some forms of this allergy can even cause almost instant death (by a process called anaphylaxis), but the vast majority of people take antibiotics for a week or 10 days or even longer without suffering any adverse consequences.

With this kind of track record—a superb benefit-to-risk ratio—it is no wonder that both doctors and patients have come to trust antibiotics as a great treatment for symptoms like cough, sore throat, fever, and earache. The first problem with this approach, however, is that antibiotics are useless for most of the pathogens that cause these symptoms. Take the average sore throat that afflicts school-aged children, for example. The poor 10-year-old girl suffers in agony every time she swallows. Her fever soars to 102°F and she develops a blotchy red rash on her body, a white coating on her tongue, and flushed cheeks. She feels miserable and cannot go to school. Her mother takes her to the pediatrician, who takes the tongue depressor, tells her to open her mouth and say "Ahh," and sees the red throat typical of acute infectious pharyngitis. The pediatrician notices a bit of pus oozing from the girl's tonsils. He calls the rash "scarleptiform"[9] and declares the combination of the pus on the tonsils and this type of rash to be characteristic of strep infection. The pediatrician prescribes a 1-week course of antibiotics. He may also swab the back of the girl's throat to obtain a sample for a throat culture and/or perform a rapid strep test to see if in fact the streptococcus bacteria are growing in her throat.

The problem with all of this is that most sore throats in 10-year-old children are caused by viruses,[10] not bacteria like strep, and antibiotics have absolutely no effect on viruses. What the pediatrician should do is to prescribe antibiotics only if the rapid strep test is positive. If it isn't, he should check the results of the throat culture a day or two later and if that is positive, then prescribe antibiotics. What he should never do is prescribe antibiotics without a positive result from either the rapid test or throat culture, or both. But unfortunately, this is what doctors do all too often. The reason is in part confirmation bias. Doctors believe they can tell the difference between bacterial and viral infections when they see pus on the tonsils and blotchy red rashes on the skin. They have seen children with pus on their tonsils and blotchy red rashes get better after taking antibiotics. Hence, every time they see these things, their belief that they are caused by a bacterial infection is confirmed and they take the "logical" action of prescribing a Z-Pak[11] In fact, one study showed that between 1997 and 2010, 60% of adults received an antibiotic for a sore throat, substantially more than the 10% who should have.[12]

Of course, the fact is that doctors cannot distinguish bacterial from viral pharyngitis merely by looking in the throat or at the skin, or by any other aspect of the physical exam. When doctors examine patients with a sore throat, make a diagnosis, and then obtain the results of a throat culture, studies have shown that the doctor's ability to correctly diagnose viral versus bacterial infection is no better than chance.[13] Despite the fact that these studies have been published in important journals that doctors read, some still insist that they can tell the difference. Now we do not mean to minimize doctors' abilities to figure things out on the basis of an examination. It is sometimes dazzling to watch a cardiologist listen to a person's heart and correctly tell exactly which valve is malfunctioning or a neurologist perform an examination and determine exactly where in the brain a tumor is sitting. More often than not, sophisticated follow-up tests like echocardiograms and MRIs confirm what the cardiologist and neurologist determined from the examination. But in the case of the cause of a sore throat, only the throat culture can reveal whether it is strep or one of a multitude of viruses that cause pharyngitis, rash, fever, and coated tongues.

The problem of antibiotic overprescription is rampant throughout medicine. In a recent study published in the *Journal of the American Medical Association (JAMA)*, investigators from Harvard Medical School reported that about 70% of people who go to the doctor because they have acute bronchitis get a prescription for an antibiotic.[14] What should that rate have been? Zero. No one should get antibiotics for acute bronchitis because those medications have been shown over and over again to be ineffective for that condition. Acute bronchitis goes away on its own in about 3 weeks at most whether or not antibiotics are prescribed. For about the last 40 years various federal and professional agencies have been trying to hammer home that point, but doctors have not changed their prescribing habits at all. Patients who demand antibiotics are often blamed for this problem. According to this scenario, doctors who know better are simply afraid to say no to their patients, supposedly fearing they will go elsewhere. While that may be true, it is also the case the doctors just do not always follow the scientific evidence. Instead, they opt for what custom and their own beliefs teach them.

More ominously, it is clearly not the case that unnecessary prescribing of antibiotics is harmless.[15] First, bacteria are capable of mutating very rapidly. Mutations that cause changes in actual physical characteristics in humans and other mammals generally take thousands of years to pass down through the generations, but changes in bacteria and viruses can occur in just one generation. Antibiotics generally work by targeting a process in bacteria that involves their genes and proteins. Rapid mutation means that bacteria can quickly develop variants of these genes and proteins that are no longer sensitive to antibiotics, a phenomenon called *resistance*. Diseases that have been easily cured with antibiotics, like gonorrhea, are now more difficult to treat because strains of the bacteria have evolved that are resistant.[16] Tuberculosis is another infectious disease for which the responsible bacteria have developed widespread resistance. Every time we give someone antibiotics we create the scenario for antibiotic resistance to develop. Dr. Tom Frieden, director of the U.S. Centers for Disease Control and Prevention (CDC), recently pointed out that antibiotic resistance causes an estimated minimum of 2 million illnesses and 23,000 deaths per year in the United States.[17] The CDC listed 17 drug-resistant bacteria and one fungus as representing drug-resistant pathogens in 2013.[18]

The second reason that antibiotic overprescription is not benign is that our bodies are colonized with thousands of different kinds of bacteria that cause us absolutely no harm and in many cases inhibit the growth of other, disease-causing bacteria. Overuse of antibiotics kills the beneficial bacteria, allowing pathogenic strains to flourish. This is one of the reasons that the awful gastrointestinal disease caused by the bacterium commonly called *C. difficile* is becoming such a problem—too many people are using antibiotics who should not because they really have viral, not bacterial, infections.

Despite the fact that doctors are taught in medical school that antibiotics don't kill viruses and that overprescribing them is harmful, inappropriate antibiotic prescription remains a rampant problem. Donnelly and colleagues from the University of Alabama at Birmingham looked at data from 126 million adults who had gone to the emergency room with an upper respiratory infection (URI).[19] Despite the fact that the great majority of URIs are viral illnesses—mostly colds—a whopping 61% of them were given a prescription for an antibiotic. This led the authors of the study to conclude that "the proportion of adult ARTI [acute respiratory tract infection] patients receiving antibiotics in U.S. EDs [emergency departments] is inappropriately high."[20] In another study, patients with acute bronchitis—a type of lower respiratory illness that is, as we pointed out earlier, almost always caused by viruses—were randomized to receive the non-steroidal anti-inflammatory drug ibuprofen, an antibiotic, or a placebo.[21] The authors of the study pointed out that bronchitis is "one of the most common reasons for visits to primary care" and that "most patients with bronchitis receive antibiotics." Nevertheless, the study findings were that all three groups did equally well, getting better in about a week and a half regardless of whether they received ibuprofen, an antibiotic, or no active drug. Even among hospitalized patients, about 30% of antibiotic use is unnecessary.[22] The problem is becoming so dire that Jeremy Farrar, the director of the United Kingdom's largest medical research organization, the Wellcome Trust, recently stated, "This [the use of antibiotics] is getting to a tipping point. . . . What we will see is people increasingly failing treatment, increasingly spending longer in hospital, patients getting sicker and having complications and dying"[23]

The Big Fat Diet Debate

Sometimes, confirmation bias can affect an entire scientific field, as seems to be the case with the long-standing warning that eating foods with high fat content increases the risk for cardiovascular disease. A troubling May 2014 article published in *The Wall Street Journal* suggests that confirmation bias has influenced generations of scientists, doctors, nutritionists, and public health experts to repeat the same bad advice over and over again.[24] The article by Nina Teicholz, author of *The Big Fat Surprise: Why Butter, Meat and Cheese Belong in a Healthy Diet*, traces this long-held insistence—that eating foods rich in saturated fats increases the risk for heart attacks and strokes—to the work of Ancel Benjamin Keys, a scientist who worked at the University of Minnesota in the 1950s. Keys published results from a large, multi-country study that seemed to show that high-fat diets were associated with elevated serum cholesterol levels, which were known to be associated with increased rates of atherosclerotic heart disease and heart attacks. "Dr. Keys was formidably persuasive," Teicholz writes, "and, through sheer force of will, rose to the top of the nutrition world—even gracing the cover of Time magazine—for relentlessly championing the idea that saturated fats raise cholesterol and, as a result, cause heart attacks." Teicholz lists a number of significant scientific problems with the way in which Keys and his group conducted their studies and analyzed their data, but Keys's work captured the attention of scientists and the public alike. In one of his papers he boldly asserted the following:

> The high frequency of coronary heart disease among American men, especially in middle age, is not found among many other populations, notably among Japanese in Japan and Bantu in South Africa. Experimental, theoretical, and epidemiologic evidence implicates the diet, and especially the fats in the diet, in these differences. The search for other factors so far has been unsuccessful.
>
> It seems probable that the more common fats of the American diet, when eaten in large amounts as is often the case in the United States, may contribute to the production of relative hypercholesterolemia and so to atherogenesis. Further, there is suggestive evidence that fatty meals may induce hypercoagulability of the blood and inhibition of fibrinolysis.[25]

The idea of fat clogging up the tiny coronary arteries that feed oxygen to the heart muscle was easy to grasp. Several studies ensued that seemed to further show that low-fat diets protected against heart attacks, and once again even though these studies now seem fatally flawed, the idea that eating fat causes heart disease became so embedded that scientists saw proof of its validity wherever they looked. Soon, we all believed that eggs and steak were veritable poisons. The American Heart Association began recommending that we limit our intake of saturated fats and everyone started substituting trans-fat-laden margarine for butter.

It now appears that all of this might have been one enormous manifestation of confirmation bias. In a recent paper published in the *Annals of Internal Medicine*, Rajiv Chowdhury of the University of Cambridge in the United Kingdom and colleagues analyzed the data from 32 studies involving 530,525 study participants and concluded, "Current evidence does not clearly support cardiovascular guidelines that encourage high consumption of polyunsaturated fatty acids and low consumption of total saturated fats."[26] Using a statistical method called meta-analysis,[27] these authors found that taking all the studies together that have been done in this area there is no evidence that eating saturated fats increases the risk for heart disease.[28] The truth was there all along, but apparently scientists were so convinced that the original hypothesis was correct that they consistently made mistakes in both study design and in the interpretation of results in order to confirm what they believed to be the truth.[29] None of this was scientific fraud. This is not a case of scientists making up data or faking results. Rather, if the Chowdhury et al. findings hold up, then we will have witnessed one of the great examples of confirmation bias affecting science and public health policy of all time. Teicholz goes on in her article to assert that the recommendation to eat less fat has led to increased carbohydrate consumption, which in turn has increased the rate of diabetes. Now, according to a randomized clinical trial, it turns out that eating a low-carbohydrate diet may be better for weight loss and cardiovascular disease risk reduction, including lowering cholesterol and triglyceride levels, than a low-fat diet.[30]

No doubt we will read a great deal more about this issue in coming months and years. The proponents of low-fat diets will probably not agree too easily that they have been wrong for the last 50 plus years.

There may be other health risks to eating too much fat, including increasing the rates of some forms of cancer. The Chowdhury meta-analysis will likely be challenged: such analyses always require that the investigators make important decisions, including which studies to include in the overall database and which statistical tests to use. Those decisions are always open to challenge.

Ironically, even scientists who conduct meta-analyses can fall into the confirmation bias trap. Felicity A. Goodyear-Smith of the University of Auckland noticed that two research groups consistently came to opposite conclusions after conducting meta-analyses of the recommendation that doctors screen patients for depression. One group routinely found that such screening is effective in identifying people with depression and reducing the rates of depression among them, and the other group found that screening for depression is ineffective. When Goodyear-Smith and her colleagues looked at the individual studies included in each of the meta-analyses, they found that each of the groups tended to include in their analyses only those studies that supported their point of view. The respective groups found problems with the methodology of studies that did not support their point of view, and they felt justified excluding those studies from the analysis. Goodyear-Smith et al. hypothesize that "authors may have a belief of what the outcome of their meta-analysis will be before they start, and that this belief may guide choices that are made on the way which may impact their review's results. This is a form of confirmation bias."[31]

If in the end, however, the reports of Chowdhury et al. that challenge the high-fat diet proscription hold up, the overall result will undoubtedly be to confuse the public. For some of us, the thought that it is now okay to eat eggs, butter, liver, and whole milk products is not far from being told that it is safe to consume arsenic. The stern advice that we eat less sugar that is rapidly replacing the low-fat recommendations will be challenged as well. The question then becomes: how are we supposed to figure out who is right and what is safe to eat? We have no easy answer for this conundrum because it rests in the nature of human psychology (i.e., the tendency to confirmation bias) and scientific progress (the constant production of new data and results, some of which inevitably challenge what has previously been thought to be correct). It is unlikely in our view that most of us will ever become scientifically sophisticated enough to spot errors in the medical literature when they first occur. Even some of the world's top scientists failed to see the problems in Keys's original work. The solution will have to come from better reporting of scientific results, and this will mean improved behavior by both scientists and the media. Scientists believe in their work, as they should, but must be more cautious about how they explain things to the media. Right now, in order to gain market share, medical schools and teaching hospitals rush to publicize new results as quickly as they can. Forbearance would be a good trait to adopt in these cases. The media often latch onto anything that sounds novel or controversial, thrusting it into our attention prematurely and then failing to acknowledge when studies are not entirely conclusive or when new findings contradict old ones.

That's My Story and I'm Sticking to It

Now that we have established that everyone is prone to confirmation bias, we want to explore why confirmation bias is so steadfast. Experiments have shown quite clearly how stubbornly resistant our minds are to change, even when the original evidence we used to come to a conclusion was flimsy and new evidence completely invalidates what we believe. In a famous experiment, Craig A. Anderson, Mark R. Lepper, and Lee Ross of Stanford University told subjects that the success or failure of firefighters could be predicted by their scores on what they called the Risky-Conservative Choice Test (RCC Test). Some of the students were given examples in which a high score predicted success, and others were given examples in which high scores predicted failure, but either way the test was actually completely fictitious. Yet even after the research subjects were debriefed and told that the RCC test is totally bogus, in subsequent experiments they still maintained a belief in a relationship between the RCC test and likelihood of firefighter success. The investigators themselves seemed somewhat amazed at the outcome of the experiment, even though it confirmed their hypothesis:

> In sum, the results strongly support the hypothesis that even after the initial evidential basis for their beliefs has been totally refuted, people fail to make appropriate revisions in those beliefs. That subjects' theories survived virtually intact is particularly impressive

when one contrasts the minimal nature of the evidential base from which subjects' initial beliefs were derived (i.e., two "data points"), with the decisiveness of the discrediting to which the evidence was subjected. In everyday experience, our intuitive theories and beliefs are sometimes based on just such inconclusive data, but challenges to such beliefs and the formative data for those beliefs are rarely as decisive as the discrediting procedures employed in this study.[32]

We do not of course mean to imply that maintaining one's theories, beliefs, and positions is always an unreasonable thing to do. Obviously, a hasty willingness to change one's mind can cause havoc in an individual's life, to an organization, or even a whole country. Very often, sticking with a course of action, even when there are "bumps in the road," is exactly the right thing to do.

What we are talking about here is not a recommendation for changing one's mind at the drop of a hat but rather the need to constantly evaluate evidence. Even when "staying the course" is the chosen path, we should still carefully examine the evidence and not turn a blind eye to it. What Anderson and colleagues and others have discovered, however, is that we are prone to develop beliefs quickly and on the basis of flimsy evidence. Then, once these beliefs are laid down, confirmation bias sets in so that everything we see next is now twisted to conform to the original belief. The doctor who needlessly prescribes antibiotics thinks he is seeing a pattern of sore throat, fever, rash, and general malaise that he believes he has seen respond to antibiotics before. Hence, for him prescribing antibiotics is fully in accord with a theory he thinks is based on experience. Similarly, the scientists who insisted for so many years that high-fat diets raise cholesterol levels and increase the risk for heart attacks had that notion so ingrained in their minds that they continuously designed experiments and interpreted data that "confirmed" the hypothesis without recognizing that what they were doing was perpetuating the same error.

Well, If That Actress Has a Gun . . .

So far, we have discussed individual susceptibility to confirmation bias, but perhaps even more ominous is the way the bias can commandeer whole groups to fall for scientifically incorrect ideas. Research shows that groups of people are just as prone as individuals to exhibit bias in the way they interpret information that is presented to them on an issue.[33] Recently, a friend who knows about Jack's interest in science denial sent him a Facebook post that included a picture of a famous actress sprawled out in a provocative pose declaring that she and her husband have guns at home. The post (see figure 2) was made by a group called the Heartland Institute, a conservative think tank that defends cigarette smokers, prides itself on promoting "skepticism" about climate change, and opposes gun control laws. The post—whose accuracy we have been unable to confirm—was followed by many comments applauding the actress for her stance.[34]

Here is Jack's posted response:

> Unfortunately, here I disagree with Heartland. Even if it is true that Angelina Jolie believes she and her family are safer if there is a gun in her home, that belief is incorrect. The risk of a famous actress, or anyone else for that matter, who lives in her home being killed or seriously injured by that gun is many times higher than the chance that she will ever get to shoot an intruder. In fact, if an intruder does

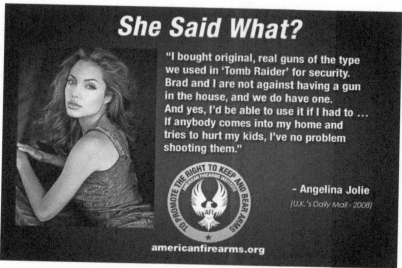

FIGURE 2 This image of the prominent actor Angelina Jolie from the British newspaper *Daily Mail* was also posted on social media by the Heartland Institute. It quotes her supporting the incorrect notion that personal gun ownership is effective protection against home invaders.

enter someone's home, a gun owner is more likely to be killed than a non-gun owner because most burglars do not wish to shoot anyone and only do so if they are threatened by someone with a gun. People who bring guns into their homes do not, of course, believe that anyone in their house will ever accidentally shoot someone or that they or a family member will ever get angry enough to shoot someone or depressed enough to shoot themselves. This is classic denial. In fact, the rates of family domestic gun violence are far higher, even among well-educated and seemingly happy families, than are the rates of home intrusion. This has nothing to do with one's right to bear arms, which is protected by the second amendment. Rather, it has to do with educating the American public that owning a gun for protection is not safe and not protection.

Immediately after this came a flood of comments such as "typical liberal drivel!! And long winded too!" and "You are a f—ing idiot." Jack tried again with some facts:

> You might try to have a look at empirical studies done on this subject. You will find that having a gun at home is a health risk. I am not debating the Second Amendment here, which absolutely protects your right to own a gun. Whether you choose to own one or not is a choice that, if you look at the data, is not supported.

The responses to this were things like "Why don't you just slap them or ask them nicely to leave while I shoot 'em?" and "If they were about to rape you, you could urinate on them. What is wrong with you?? Lolol" and

> Jack, you are an idiot. If you don't believe in guns. Then don't have guns. As for me and most educated people, we have guns. I feel safer when I carry concealed and I feel safer at home. If someone breaks into your home, dial 911 and hope that the police get there before you get shot. Someone that is willing to break into an occupied home, is willing to shoot those occupants. I would rather be judged by 12 than carried by 6.

Jack even provided references to the published scientific literature to back up his claims. But what is fascinating is that none of his interlocutors from the Heartland site addressed the data. Although the great majority of studies examining the safety of private gun ownership have reached the conclusion that it is unsafe, there are a handful of published studies with conflicting data. That is always true in any scientific arena. These are not easy studies to do. One has to troll through large data sets to identify (a) who has a gun, (b) who was shot with their own gun or a gun owned by someone with whom they reside, (c) who was the victim of an armed home invasion, and (d) what was the outcome of the invasion. Merging data sets like these can be a daunting task, especially since there are inevitably missing data, such as data that need to be excluded because they make no sense (e.g., an entry for a 400-year-old man) or data that are unclear (what exactly was the relationship of the person shot to the person who owned the gun?). There are also always issues about what time frame to pick, which region of the country, how to ensure that the sample is representative of the general population of gun owners (no skewing in terms of age, sex, socioeconomic status, etc.), and which statistical methods to use to analyze the data.

The leading academic voice supporting the notion that firearms are necessary for self-defense is Gary Kleck, a professor of criminology at Florida State University. Kleck is a respected and often-quoted academic who has done extensive research and writing on gun control. He insists that the evidence shows that guns are often used by private citizens in the prevention of crimes and that laws restricting gun ownership increase the risk for gun violence. Perhaps his most famous assertion is that 2.5 million Americans use guns to defend themselves against attackers every year.[35] This assertion has aroused derision on the part of a host of other academics who insist that the research methodology used by Kleck and coauthor Marc Gertz is completely invalid. Harvard's David Hemenway, for example, asserts that the number is grossly inflated.[36] The Kleck and Gertz study was done by a telephone survey of a relatively small number of people whose responses were then projected to a national annual number. There is reason to believe that many people who participate in such telephone surveys misremember or even falsify what really happened and also that the extrapolation of the results from the small sample to a national statistic may have been inexact.

On balance, the weight of data showing that private gun ownership is unsafe is incontrovertible. But the gun enthusiasts who confronted Jack could have brought up Kleck's work and tried to base their argument on published data. The exchange would then have moved away from epithets and sloganeering. But nothing like that happened. Jack tried several times to push the data aspect, each time flatly stating what the studies show. He deliberately avoided attacking the gun proponents on a personal level, getting angry at being called an "idiot" and "a moron," or trying to defend his intelligence. Each time he pointed out the data, however, the opposition seemed to get even angrier and more dogmatic. Indeed, they seemed to be having a good time. This may seem odd to some; after all, we were talking about people getting shot and killed. Whether you think you are going to shoot an armed burglar or rapist or your child is going to find your gun and shoot him- or herself, there is absolutely nothing entertaining about the outcome of gun violence. But the impression one gets when reading the Facebook exchange is of a group rallying itself into a fervor of righteous indignation and solidarity.

The impression Jack got from this is that the gun proponents who responded to his data-driven overtures extracted only what they already believed. Jack said, "Studies show that a gun in the home is more likely to be used to shoot its owner or a family member than an intruder," and they replied, "You idiot." No one said, "Let me think about those facts you are bringing up." No one asked for further information or clarification of the data. The assumption was simply made that Jack is a liberal who is trying to take away their Second Amendment rights. This was a clear lesson in the reality of confirmation bias. Gun proponents believe that their opponents are completely naïve about the reality of violence in the world, live in an ivory tower, are privileged and elitist, and would not hold to their beliefs if they themselves were challenged by someone with a gun. They seem to believe that home invasions by armed intruders are rampant (they are actually quite rare) and that because they themselves supposedly know how to store their guns safely and educate their children about how to use them properly none of the scientific data about the dangers of having a gun at home apply to them. No matter what Jack said, these beliefs were continuously reaffirmed. Jack's foray into the Heartland reified what the gun proponents already believed and gave them a communal activity they seemed to enjoy. In the end, Jack probably succeeded in making them even more convinced that guns are not only safe but also necessary to own. The group dynamic of defeating a common enemy simply made this confirmation firmer.

Michael Shermer, the provocative editor of *Skeptic* magazine, recently wrote that he once believed that gun control violated his libertarian principles:

> Then I read the science on guns and homicides, suicides and accidental deaths.... Although the data to convince me that we need some gun-control measures were there all along, I had ignored them because they didn't fit my creed.... In several recent debates with economist John R. Lott, Jr., author of *More Guns, Less Crime*, I saw a reflection of my former self in the cherry picking and data mining of studies to suit ideological convictions.[37]

This is quite a confession from someone who has based his career on rigorously sticking with the evidence, even when it disconfirms very popular notions. Yet even Michael Shermer acknowledges the power of confirmation bias in making us ignore what we are afraid will contradict what we want to believe. How much more difficult to flaunt the confirmation bias will it be for those of us not as devoted to evidence as Michael Shermer?

Who Says Emotions Are Harmless?

In his book *Social Networks and Popular Understanding of Science and Health*, Brian G. Southwell explores many of the ways in which group membership strengthens an individual's tendency to adhere to confirmation bias. He points to extensive research showing that when people are provoked to a heightened emotional state they are more likely to share information. When that state is an unpleasant one, like fear or anger, emotionally aroused people come together to seek comfort from each other. "Much of the discussion we seek with others in moments of elevated emotion," Southwell writes, "is not necessarily focused on new factual information sharing as much as it is focused on reassurance, coping with stress, and ritualistic bonding."[38] The purpose of groups like Heartland is not to help people understand both sides of an issue or to be able to come to a reasoned position about an important health decision.

Membership in such groups may begin with someone—let us call her Jane—who is not sure how she feels about having a gun. In fact, she doesn't own one herself. Jane is, however, a cigarette smoker who despite trying everything from self-help groups to hypnotism to medication has been unable to quit. Every day, it seems, she is confronted with accusations that she is weak-willed for not being able to stop smoking, that she is poisoning herself and others, and that no one really wants her around. She is ordered outside whenever she wants—perhaps *needs* is a better way to put it—to smoke. That makes her feel as if the whole world is shunning her. Cigarette smokers as a group tend to have higher rates of depression than the general population as it is.[39] Jane's level of self-confidence cannot be helped by constantly being told that there are many public places in which she is not welcome if she is going to smoke. Sometimes Jane feels terrible about herself and other times she gets angry. After all, she is a citizen and has rights just like everyone else. One day she reads an article in her local newspaper about an organization called Heartland that defends the rights of cigarette smokers. In fact, Heartland defends people from that clique of self-righteous, wealthy liberals who are always trying to make everyone's life miserable by telling them that everything we do is going to kill us. We are not supposed to smoke, drink, eat the foods we like, drive our cars, or have guns. And for the privilege of all these rules we have to pay higher and higher taxes.

Jane starts following Heartland on social media. She finds it comforting to interact with so many people who feel similarly abused and neglected. She finds out that not only are there many other people who smoke, there are people who do not feel there is anything wrong with it. These people also warn that the liberals who want to make her feel like an outlaw for smoking also don't care if she gets shot during a burglary or raped. They say that everyone has a right to smoke and to own a gun and that all the handwringing about climate warming is just so much hot air (pun intended). Soon, Jane begins to worry for the first time that her house could be broken into any day. What would she do? She would be completely defenseless. There would be no way to protect herself or her children from one of those crazy maniacs you hear about all the time on the news who shoot people just because they feel like it. Jane buys a gun.[40]

When Jane reads the comments of someone like Jack, all of her anger is aroused. For her, Jack is not really just trying to start a calm discussion about scientific studies about gun ownership. Everything he says is completely reminiscent of every hectoring liberal telling her she is a bad person. His every word confirms her belief that Jack is exactly the kind of person against whom she must defend herself. After years of being told each time she lights up or throws out her garbage that she is contributing to the destruction of the world, Jane now joins her online social group in gleefully attacking Jack.

There are of course a number of mechanisms that go into Jane's attitude about guns and her decision to join a group like Heartland. She believes that there is a conspiracy against her and the members of her new group, for example. But here we wish to point out that even though Jane has never read any of the scientific papers for or against gun ownership, she has found a home among a group of total believers. Thus, the Internet, which is supposed to provide us with all the information we need to make rational decisions and choices, has actually reified an irrational idea in Jane's mind and prevented her from even trying to consider disconfirming evidence for her point of view. Furthermore, Jane came to the conclusion that Heartland's followers must be right about gun ownership when she was in a heightened emotional or "affective" state. Strong evidence shows that people are more prone to believe what they are told whenever they are in such a state, whether it is a positive or negative one. That is, regardless of whether we are deliriously happy or morbidly sad, we are likely to believe what we are being told. "Affect," writes Paul Slovic, the eminent behavioral psychologist, "is a strong conditioner of preference."[41] This is why politicians know that they need to get their audience emotionally aroused before trying to convince them.

Another aspect of Jane's adoption of the pro-gun ownership hypothesis is her feeling of dread regarding potential home invaders. Even though the evidence does not support the likelihood that most people will actually ever experience such an event, gun proponents paint vivid pictures of the instances in which a home invasion by armed intruders has occurred. This is, of course, reinforced by what we see on television and in movies. As Slovic puts it, "Perceptions of risk and society's responses to risk were strongly linked to the degree to which a hazard evoked feelings of dread."[42] Most important for our understanding of confirmation bias is that beliefs laid down during times of heightened emotion, especially those involving terror and dread, are highly durable and resistant to disconfirmation. Every time we re-experience those emotions, the belief is also brought immediately to mind.[43] It is much easier for someone to induce us to summon up a feeling of dread than to get us to work deliberatively through the data on whether or not there is a protective advantage of having a gun at home. So what we learn when we are emotionally aroused is thereafter hard to shake.

Southwell stresses that people who lack self-confidence cannot be expected to contradict the ideas of a group that comforts them:

> We know that people are not particularly likely to share information they do not think they understand. Absent direct encouragement to challenge or engage with scientific ideas, such as research on medical innovations or biotechnology, many people will silently defer to those they see as relatively expert. . . . Individuals who feel as though they can grasp key ideas are more likely to subsequently share those ideas with others.[44]

The question, of course, then becomes, how can we boost the confidence of individuals like our fictitious Jane so that they can grasp enough about a scientific discussion to make a reasoned decision? Without doing so, per Southwell, we are left with individuals who will make up their minds first on the basis of the emotional aspects of an issue, like fear and anger, and then see everything that is subsequently said about the issue as directly confirming what they believe.

It's All in Your Brain

What is it that we concentrate on when we become swayed by a group like Heartland that promulgates ideas that defy scientific evidence? Does the group actually change our minds about the issues at hand or is it the social affiliation that induces joining in? How does the fixed conviction that is so ferociously defended by the confirmation bias actually initiated? In a very elegant experiment, Gregory S. Berns and his colleagues at Emory University sought to understand whether when individuals follow an incorrect group consensus it is because they are making an active decision to go along with the group or because their perception of the issue has been altered.[45] In this experiment, social conformity was associated with a decrease in activation of the frontal lobe, the part of the brain that controls reason and other executive functions, and an increase in activity in the parietal and occipital lobes, regions of the brain where perceptions are formed. The conclusion from these data is that social conformity is not a conscious decision but rather it is based on actual alterations in how we see reality. When subjects did act independently of the group in the Berns et al experiment, there was more activation in the amygdala. The amygdala, as discussed in the last chapter, is buried deep in one of the more primitive parts of the brain and has been shown to be especially important in the recognition of danger and the psychological and physical manifestations of fear. Our conclusion from this, which differs somewhat from Berns's interpretation, is that defying your group is a frightening proposition that must hold the promise of some reward in order to be tenable. In fact, other studies have shown that a decrease in biased thinking is associated with a decrease in amygdala activity.[46] Somehow, we need to reduce the fear that is understandably associated with changing one's mind.

The Berns study of brain activation patterns suggests that people do not become affiliated with anti-science groups simply because they are lonely and want to "belong." Rather, the way they perceive an issue is actually altered. This change in brain activity solidifies the new beliefs as part of a fixed biological structure that then resists further alteration. To now defy the group's beliefs activates the amygdala and causes fear. Confirmation bias, then, reinforces the new safety of believing in the group's point of view.

Evaluating a belief that we are sure is true, and challenging that belief, even to the point of disconfirmation, is an exhausting process. To do it well, we need to suppress our emotions and try to think as rationally and clearly as possible. To behavioral economists, this means favoring System 2 over System 1. As we discuss throughout this book, these two systems represent a rough distinction between the more sophisticated and recently evolved System 2 centers of our brains located mainly in the prefrontal cortex (PFC), sometimes referred to as the rule-based brain, and the more emotional and primitive System 1 centers, located in what is referred to as the limbic cortex, also called the associative brain.

Lest we leap to the conclusion that the associative brain is somehow inferior to the rule-based brain, it is important to acknowledge that the former is necessary for intuition, fantasy, creativity, and imagination.[47] Without it, we would probably have no art and no empathy. Humans are the only truly altruistic species,[48] and without an associative brain we would not witness individuals giving money to homeless people on the street when there is absolutely no possibility of material reward for their generosity. The rule-based brain can be the driver of rather dry behaviors, like deliberation, formal analysis, and strategic planning. It is, however, the part of the brain we need to use if we are going to make decisions that are evidence-based and not tainted by emotion.

It is also not the case that the preferential use of the rule-oriented, or System 2, brain indicates that a person is smart. Cognitive ability, including intelligence, is unrelated to the tendency toward confirmation bias.[49] Smart people, including Nobel Prize–winning scientists, are entirely capable of seeing only what they already believe.

Moreover, as Daniel Kahneman and his colleagues have shown through extensive research, the more tired and depleted we are, the more prone we are to relying on easier sources to make decisions and therefore committing confirmation biases. The human brain is an incredible energy-consuming organ, burning glucose for fuel at a higher rate than any other part of the body. When we are tired, hungry, depressed, or distracted it is harder to spend the energy and therefore our mental processes default to the easiest method of reaching a decision. This usually means employing only limbic, or System 1, parts of the brain and therefore leaving us prone to committing errors by using shortcuts like confirmation bias.

Confirmation Bias: As Good as Eating a Candy Bar

Using confirmation bias to make decisions may actually make us feel good in the way that people experience the positive effects of alcohol or opiates. Although again an oversimplification, there is a "reward" pathway in the brain that runs from a structure in the brainstem called the ventral tegmental area (VTA) to one deep in the lower part of the brain called the nucleus accumbens (NA, NAc, or NAcc). The pathway releases the neurotransmitter dopamine whenever we (or almost any animal) anticipates or experiences a rewarding or pleasurable stimulus. Studies have confirmed, for example, that this pathway is activated and dopamine released into synapses (the spaces between brain cells or neurons) whenever we sip an alcoholic beverage. Alcoholics, unfortunately, drink to the point that the pathway becomes exhausted and dopamine depleted, so that they need to drink ever-increasing amounts to get the same effect. But for most people, an occasional drink activates the pathway and creates a warm, pleasurable feeling. Research also indicates that the NAc is activated before making a risky financial choice.[50] This reinforces the thrill of investing that many in the financial world experience.

According to Noreena Hertz, author of *Eyes Wide Open: How to Make Smart Decisions in a Confusing World,* "We actually get a dopamine rush when we find confirming data, similar to the one we get if we eat chocolate, have sex, or fall in love. Having jumped to a particular conclusion, we focus on information that supports it, and ignore everything that contradicts or doesn't conform to our initial analysis."[51]

Once again it is important to remember that confirmation bias, like all of the psychological mechanisms we identify that motivate denial of scientific evidence in this book, is by no means "irrational" even though it can lead to incorrect ideas. Rather, confirmation bias is a part of the way the human brain naturally works. Indeed, we are rewarded for using confirmation bias by the powerful actions of dopamine in the pleasure centers of our brains. In other words, it feels good to "stick to our guns" even if we are wrong. When understood in terms of human brain physiology in this way, getting a person to even momentarily shun what she believes in order to attend carefully to potentially disconfirming evidence requires some guarantee that the risk of doing so will produce a reward at least equal to the one she will get by succumbing to confirmation bias. Research needs to be done, then, to determine what rewards will be adequate to motivate adults to look at the data with an open mind. Is that reward based in an altruistic feeling of doing the right thing for other people? Would those who are vehemently opposed to GMOs agree to at least consider the possibility that GMOs are safe if doing so would make them feel that they are potentially helping starving children in Africa survive or preventing Asian children from going blind? Or perhaps the reward would come from securely joining a new group. Can a person rigidly against vaccination see a possible reward—and its concomitant dopamine surge—if he is shown that changing his mind would put him into contact with a large group of parents, scientists, and doctors whose main interest is in protecting children from dying from preventable diseases like measles and diphtheria?

Of course people vary in how much risk they are willing to take—including how much risk they are willing to take in changing their minds from a fixed belief to one that is based on new evidence. Interestingly, some of this interpersonal variability may be caused by differences in two genes, one of which is active in the dopamine system.[52] We inherit different forms of the same gene from our parents and each form is called an allele. There are five proteins in the brain that act as receptors for the neurotransmitter dopamine, one of which is called the DRD4 receptor. The gene that encodes this receptor has a variant called the 7-repeat allele, and people who are carriers of it take 25% more risk than individuals without the 7-repeat allele of the DRD4 gene. Hence, how much of a boost a person gets from changing or staying with a belief could be in part a function of what kind of dopamine receptor genes he or she has inherited. Of course, other genes are also involved, including genes involved in the serotonin receptor system,[53] as are a host of nongenetic factors. Despite these individual differences, some basics of brain biology and function can demonstrate just how naturally human the tendency toward confirmation bias is.

Just Give Me the Facts

If confirmation bias is so ingrained in our very humanity, how can we attempt to disarm it? We do at least know what does *not* work. Merely giving people facts that contradict their beliefs is not sufficient to disconfirm those beliefs. In fact, evidence suggests that such a strategy can actually reinforce confirmation bias because people tend to be much gentler when evaluating evidence that confirms their beliefs than when evaluating contradictory evidence. There is almost no such thing as a scientific paper without some flaws. In fact, it is customary in the final section of scientific papers for the authors to list all of the limitations of their study. They may acknowledge that their sample size was rather small, that the subjects in their study were not completely representative of the general American population (e.g., most of them were from a single socioeconomic class), or that blood samples from the research subjects were frozen and stored rather than being tested immediately.

The conclusion the authors reach from this scientific mea culpa is that "more research needs to be done." Now, if the authors can identify flaws in their study even though they clearly believe in the importance of the work, it should not be difficult for independent readers to find infelicities as well. But if the study supports our ideas then we tend to gloss over such shortcomings, whereas if it contradicts them we attack with ruthless vigor, picking apart every detail possible.

Charles G. Lord of Texas Christian University and his coauthors demonstrated this point in an experiment in which they recruited undergraduates who either supported or opposed the death penalty. The students were asked to read two papers supposedly representing actual research, one that found that capital punishment is a deterrent to crime and the other that it is not. As the investigators predicted, the students who favored the death penalty rated the paper that allegedly found a deterrent effect as more credible than the one that found it does not, while the students who were against the death penalty made the opposite ratings. Thus, at the end of the experiment, rather than being brought closer together by having had the opportunity to review data on both sides of the issue, the students were actually more convinced that they were right. Lord et al. concluded that, "The net effect of such evaluations and opinion shifts was the postulated increase in attitude polarization."[54]

Proving Ourselves Wrong

There is at least one instance in which an understanding of confirmation bias has revolutionized the treatment of a medical condition. Aaron T. Beck recognized that people suffering from depression focus most on things in their environment that give them a reason to be depressed.[55] Only negative information is consumed, and anything positive is either not noticed or dismissed as unreliable. Beck developed a groundbreaking psychotherapeutic method for challenging this mode of thinking called cognitive therapy. In some ways, cognitive therapy is devoted to undermining the confirmation bias of patients with depression by restoring their ability to recognize evidence of both positive and negative things in their environments. There is even brain imaging data that suggest that cognitive therapy helps restore the ability of the prefrontal cortex to muster reason to regulate the emotional outpourings of the amygdala and other limbic structures. Today, cognitive therapy stands as one of the most effective interventions for depression and a number of other psychiatric disorders. Jack has long advocated Beck as a great candidate for a Nobel Prize.

For the most part blind application of confirmation bias commits us to maintaining mistakes that almost always ultimately result in harm. The people who think that genetically modified foods are dangerous to human health passionately believe that they are protecting everyone from huge but vaguely specified risks that are being deliberately obfuscated by large corporations and their paid scientific lackeys. Ironically, anti-GMO exponents are generally among the people most horrified by poverty and starvation and expend a great deal of effort fighting against income inequality and discrimination. They might be expected to be the very people who would wholeheartedly endorse GMOs as a way of saving the lives of millions of impoverished Africans and Asians. But at this point, explaining to them that GMO foods are in fact not dangerous and that without them millions of people stand to suffer diseases and hunger that could be averted has virtually no impact. They are adamant and organized and admit only those facts that seem to support their point of view.

The task of turning our attention to a reasonable and ongoing evaluation of evidence is daunting in the face of the power of confirmation bias. As we suggest elsewhere in this book, it will require a major shift in the way we educate children about science. This will necessarily involve turning away from memorizing facts that, however important they may be, are seen as boring and oppressive, and toward an understanding and appreciation of the scientific method and the way science operates. There are, however, some shorter term innovations that may at least be partially helpful.

In the Anderson, Lepper, and Ross experiments mentioned earlier in this chapter, the investigators also established that having people write down their reasons for coming to a conclusion abetted their future inflexibility in considering disconfirming evidence. They asked some of the research subjects who had read the information that the bogus RCC test could predict the future success or failure of a firefighter to write down how they had come to the conclusion that there is a relationship between RCC test score and success/failure. Compared to those participants who were not asked to explicitly state their thinking in written form, those subjects were less likely to change their minds after the debriefings informed them that the whole relationship was fictitious and based on nonsense rather than actual data. Being required to write down how one understands a theoretical relationship, even one that later proves to be false, thus reified the belief. The researchers speculate on this finding:

> It suggests ... an interesting potential antidote for unwarranted belief perseverance in the face of later challenge to the evidence on which our beliefs were based.
>
> Would such perseverance effects be eliminated or attenuated, for example, if subjects could be led, after debriefing, to consider explicitly the explanations that might be offered to support a contention in opposition to their initial beliefs? Alternatively, could subjects be "inoculated" against perseverance effects if they had been asked, at the outset of the study, to list all of the possible reasons they could imagine that might have produced either a positive or a negative relationship between the two variables being studied ... ?"[56]

Is there a way to engage open-minded people—at least those people who have not yet irrevocably laid down their beliefs and joined like-minded groups—in exercises in which, instead of telling them the facts, they are asked to imagine different sides of a controversy, different outcomes, and different interpretations? Neurobiologists and cognitive psychologists know that passive learning is far less efficient than learning that occurs when students are performing a task, which could include writing down their responses to various alternative scenarios. An example would be to ask GMO skeptics to write down how they would deal with evidence that such foods are not in fact harmful to human health. We would not require the participants to agree that this was the case, merely to write down what they think would happen, how they would feel, and what would be the consequences if that turned out to be correct. This is, of course, a scientifically evaluable suggestion—a testable hypothesis is that such exercises would result in people who are more open-minded and willing to at least look at the data. Hopefully, such experiments are already taking place and educators will devise schemes to introduce these ideas—if and only if they prove successful in the laboratory—to widespread public distribution. Most important, we need to challenge people to think for themselves by asking them to imagine alternative scenarios including those with which they tend to disagree. We stress that lecturing, scientists' usual method to try to rectify entrenched misconceptions, does not work. The process has to be far more interactive and iterative.

We invite our readers, then, to try this procedure in a personal experiment. Think of something you feel strongly about that you believe is supported by strong scientific evidence. Now, go to a quiet place when you are relatively free from stress or distraction and write down what you know about the arguments on the other side of your belief. Also, write down what it would take for you to change your mind. You may find that after doing this you will feel the urge to check out the data a bit more than you did in the past and to listen to alternative ideas. You may not wind up changing your mind, but either way we predict that you feel more secure in and satisfied with your point of view.

It is also important to approach people in the right way and at the right time. Because tackling the task of evaluating potentially disconfirming evidence requires a great deal of exhausting effort on the part of our prefrontal cortex, and because we cannot use electrical stimulation to activate this region of the brain on a widespread or regular basis, we need to devise ways of attracting people's attention when they are well rested and relatively open to novelty, not in states of depression or high anxiety. This is a job for advertising and marketing experts, who have perfected the art of delivering persuasive messages in ways that maximize results. We are not advocating manipulating the public, but rather borrowing what these experts in information transfer have learned to develop more successful ways of encouraging people to listen to the facts.

It will also be critically important to recognize that people hold onto their beliefs for profound emotional reasons that are reinforced by predictable activity in specific brain circuits and networks. Retaining an idea and affiliating with like-minded members of a group activates the reward centers of our brains, making us feel righteous, safe, and loved. If we are going to move people in the direction of dispassionate regard for scientific truth, we must accept the fact that their current beliefs are based on entirely understandable principles. Indeed, the confirmation bias is not a bizarre or even irrational phenomenon but rather the result of the way our brains have evolved to make sure we remain steady, cooperate with friends and associates, and are generally in a positive state so we can succeed. As Lisa Rosenbaum elegantly states in her *New England Journal of Medicine* article:

> Among those of us in the business of evidence-based risk reduction, terms such as "social values" and "group identities" may elicit a collective squirm. But developing an understanding of how such factors inform our perceptions of disease is critical to improving the health of our population. Certainly, understanding of one's risk for any disease must be anchored in facts. But if we want our facts to translate into better health, we may need to start talking more about our feelings.[57]

Indeed, if we want people to understand that owning a gun is dangerous, that stopping GMOs contributes to disease and starvation, and that overprescribing antibiotics is counterproductive, we need to empathize with the powerful emotions and brain circuits that underlie denial of these scientifically unassailable facts. We need to encourage people to write down their ideas, try to think of alternatives, and recognize when it is their emotions rather than their frontal lobes that are guiding their decisions.

As we have shown, confirmation bias can strike both groups and individuals in different but important ways. In the second part of this book, we turn to more "individual" forms of incorrect scientific beliefs, by which we mean incorrect beliefs that thrive in the individual mind, not because of group dynamics in particular. We begin with one of the most intriguing examples: the desire to attribute causality in situations of immense uncertainty.

Causality and Filling the Ignorance Gap

Coincidence obeys no laws and if it does we don't know what they are. Coincidence, if you'll permit me the simile, is like the manifestation of God at every moment on our planet. A senseless God making senseless gestures at his senseless creatures. In that hurricane, in that osseous implosion, we find communion.
—Roberto Bolaño

T HERE IS AN OLD ADAGE: "WHAT YOU DON'T KNOW CAN'T hurt you." In the science denial arena, however, this adage seems to have been recrafted to something like: "What you don't know is an invitation to make up fake science." Before it was discovered that tuberculosis is caused by a rather large bacteria called *Mycobacterium tuberculosis* it was widely believed to be the result of poor moral character. Similarly, AIDS was attributed to "deviant" lifestyles, like being gay or using intravenous drugs. When we don't know what causes something, we are pummeled by "experts" telling us what to believe. Vaccines cause autism. ECT causes brain damage. GMOs cause cancer.

Interestingly, the leap by the public to latch onto extreme theories does not extend to all branches of science. Physicists are not certain how the force of gravity is actually conveyed between two bodies. The theoretical solutions offered to address this question involve mind-boggling mathematics and seemingly weird ideas like 12 dimensional strings buzzing around the universe. But we don't see denialist theories about gravity all over the Internet. Maybe this is simply because the answer to the question does not seem to affect our daily lives one way or the other. But it is also the case that even though particle physics is no more or less complex than molecular genetics, we all believe the former is above our heads but the latter is within our purview. Nonphysicists rarely venture an opinion on whether or not dark matter exists, but lots of nonbiologists will tell you exactly what the immune system can and cannot tolerate. Even when scientific matters become a little more frightening, when they occur in some branches of science, they register rather mild attention. Some people decided that the supercollider in Switzerland called the Large Hadron Collider (LHC) might be capable of producing black holes that would suck in all of Earth. Right before the LHC was scheduled to be tested at full capacity, there were a few lawsuits filed around the world trying to stop it on the grounds that it might induce the end of the world. A few newspapers even picked up on the story. But there were no mass protests or Congressional hearings. Nobody tried to storm the LHC laboratories to stop the experiment. Scientists knew all along that the black hole prediction was mistaken. The LHC was turned on, high-energy beams of subatomic particles collided, and something called the Higgs boson (sometimes called the "God particle") was discovered. Many popular news outlets celebrated this wonderful advance in particle physics, testimony to our enduring interest in science. How different the response of the media to the claim that nuclear power will destroy the world. Scientists tell us that isn't the case, but to many their considered reassurance makes no difference at all.

Perhaps understandably, when it comes to our health, everyone is an expert, and when we don't know the cause of something we care deeply about, we can gravitate en masse to all kinds of proposals. Sometimes those theories contain a germ of plausibility to them— the idea that a mercury preservative called thimerosal that was used to preserve vaccines might be linked to autism was not entirely out of the question. It is just that careful research proved it to be wrong. But before that happened, the idea that vaccines cause autism was already ingrained in the minds of many vulnerable people, especially parents of children with autism desperately searching for answers.

Similarly, we are frightened when we get coughs and colds. Viruses are mysterious entities, so we decide that a class of medication called antibiotics is going to kill them and cure us. Although we do now have some drugs that successfully treat viral illnesses like HIV and herpes, the ones we take for what we believe are sinus infections and "bad head colds," drugs like "Z-Pak," are totally ineffective against these viral illnesses. For the most part, scientists don't know how to treat viral illnesses, and therefore the myth that common antibiotics will do the trick fills the knowledge gap. Even doctors behave as if they believe it, despite the fact that they are all taught in medical school that this is absolutely not the case. It is simply too frightening to accept the fact that we don't know what causes something or how to cure it. So why do we trust experts when they tell us that black holes are not going to suck us up but think we are the experts when we tell our doctor we must have a Z-Pak? How can we live with uncertainty, even when that uncertainty extends to scientists who have not—and never will—figure out all the answers?

In this chapter, we seek to understand why people feel the need to fill the ignorance gap. We argue that it is highly adaptive to know how to attribute causality but that people are often too quick to do so. This is another instance in which adaptive, evolutionary qualities have done us a disservice in the face of complex debates and rational thinking. In particular, people have a difficult time sitting with uncertainty and an especially hard time accepting coincidence. We consider the evidence from decades of psychological research showing people's misunderstanding of cause and effect and the elaborate coping mechanisms we have developed as a result. Finally, we suggest some ways to help us better comprehend true causality, without diminishing our ability to attribute cause when it is in fact appropriate.

What Is a Cause?

There is actually no easy answer to the question "What is a cause?" Philosophers, scientists, and economists have been arguing for centuries over what constitutes causality, and there is no reason to believe that any of these fields has a great answer to the question. The issue of causality really begins with Aristotle. Aristotle's theory of the four causes (material, formal, efficient, and final) is extremely complex and not too central here, but an aspect of Aristotle's philosophy of cause that is useful for our purposes is the notion that we do not have knowledge of something until we know its cause. Aristotle presented this notion in *Posterior Analytics,* and the concept behind it seems to describe a central inclination of human psychology. We want to know the *why* of everything. Anyone who has been around a small child has perhaps not so fond memories of the *why* game. The child will get into a mood or phase in which he or she asks "Why?" about everything you do or say. "I'm going to the grocery store," you might say, and the child will immediately ask, "Why?" "Because I need to get bananas," you might respond, and the child will immediately ask "Why?" again. "Because I like bananas in my cereal," and the child asks, "Why?" and so forth. This behavior is extremely frustrating for an adult, since at a certain point we grow tired of providing explanations for everything we are doing. However, insofar as children represent uninhibited human inclinations, the desire to know the *why* of everything is a basic human instinct. Aristotle simply formalized this intuitive notion by making it clear that we are never comfortable with our knowledge of a subject until we know the "why" behind it. Scientists may know that the MERS coronavirus is a SARS-like contagious disease spreading throughout the Middle East, but they will not stop their investigation and proclaim "knowledge" of this particular outbreak until they understand where precisely it originated.

Aristotle is often referred to as the father of science, but a lot of our scientific thoughts about causality come more directly from the British empiricists of the 18th century, especially David Hume. Hume and his contemporaries were basically obsessed with the notion of "experience" and how it generates knowledge. Accordingly, Hume found a problem with using inductive reasoning to establish causation, a not inconsequential finding since this is the fundamental way that scientists attempt to establish that something causes something else. Hume basically left us with a puzzle: if we always observe B occurring after A, we will automatically think that A causes B due to their contiguity. Hume of course notes that this perception does not mean that A is actually the cause of B. Yet he is more interested in establishing how we perceive causality than in defining what a cause truly is. In this sense, Hume's philosophy represents a kind of psychological theory. How we perceive causality will be based on temporality and contiguity, whether or not these are truly reliable ways of establishing causality. In other words, we are naturally inclined to attribute the experience of constant contiguity to causality.

In 1843, John Stuart Mill converted some of this philosophizing on causation into a more scientific process of inquiry. Mill posited five methods of induction that could lead us to understand causality. The first is the *direct method of agreement*. This method suggests that if something is a necessary cause, it must always be present when we observe the effect. For example, if we always observe that the varicella zoster virus causes chickenpox symptoms, then varicella zoster must be a necessary cause of chickenpox. We cannot observe any cases of chickenpox symptoms in which the varicella zoster virus is not present.

The second method is the *method of difference*. If two situations are exactly the same in every aspect except one, and the effect occurs in one but not the other situation, then the one aspect they do not have in common is likely to be the cause of the effect of interest. For example, if two people spent a day eating exactly the same foods except one person ate potato salad and the other did not, and one ends up with food poisoning and the other is not sick, Mill would say that the potato salad is probably the cause of the food poisoning. The third method is a simple *combination of the methods of agreement and difference*.

Mill's fourth method is the *method of residue*. In this formulation, if a range of conditions causes a range of outcomes and we have matched the conditions to the outcomes on all factors except one, then the remaining condition must cause the remaining outcome. For example, if a patient goes to his doctor complaining of indigestion, rash, and a headache, and he had eaten pizza, coleslaw, and iced tea for lunch, and we have established that pizza causes rashes and iced tea causes headaches, then we can deduce that coleslaw must cause indigestion.

The final method is the *method of concomitant variation*. In this formulation, if one property of a phenomenon varies in tandem with some property of the circumstance of interest, then that property most likely causes the circumstance. For example, if various samples of water contain the same ratio of concentrations of salt and water and the level of toxicity varies in tandem with the level of lead in the water, then it could be assumed that the toxicity level is related to the lead level and not the salt level.

Following on the heels of Mill, scientific theories of causation developed further with Karl Popper and Austin Bradford Hill. In 1965, Hill devised nine criteria for causal inference that continue to be taught in epidemiology classes around the world:

1. *Strength:* the larger the association, the more likely it is causal.
2. *Consistency:* consistent observations of suspected cause and effect in various times and places raise the likelihood of causality.
3. *Specificity:* the proposed cause results in a specific effect in a specific population.
4. *Temporality:* the cause precedes the effect in time.
5. *Biological gradient:* greater exposure to the cause leads to a greater effect.
6. *Plausibility:* the relationship between cause and effect is biologically and scientifically plausible.
7. *Coherence:* epidemiological observation and laboratory findings confirm each other.
8. *Experiment:* when possible, experimental manipulation can establish cause and effect.
9. *Analogy:* cause-and-effect relationships have been established for similar phenomena.

Some of these criteria are much more acceptable to modern epidemiologists than are others. For example, any scientist will agree that temporality is essential in proving causality. If the correct timeline of events is missing, causality cannot be established. On the other hand, criteria such as analogy and specificity are much more debated. These criteria are generally viewed as weak suggestions of causality but can by no means "prove" a cause-and-effect relationship.

If It Can Be Falsified It Might Be True

In the early 20th century, Popper defined what has come to be a central tenet of the scientific notion of causality and, more specifically, the kind of causality that becomes so difficult for nonscientists to grasp. For Popper, proving causality was the wrong goal. Instead, induction should proceed not by *proving* but by *disproving*. Popper is thus often seen as the forefather of empirical falsification, a concept central to modern scientific inquiry. Any scientific hypothesis must be falsifiable. This is why the statement "There is a God" is not a scientific hypothesis because it is impossible to disprove. The goal of scientific experimentation, therefore, is to try to disprove a hypothesis by a process that resembles experience or empirical observation. It is this line of thinking that informs the way hypothesis testing is designed in science and statistics. We are always trying to *disprove* a *null hypothesis,* which is the hypothesis that there is in fact no finding. Therefore, a scientific finding will always be a matter of rejecting the null hypothesis and never a matter of accepting the alternative hypothesis.

For example, in testing a new medication, the technical aspects of acceptable modern experimental design frame the question being asked not as "Can we prove that this new drug works?" but rather "With how much certainty can we disprove the idea that this drug does not work?" As we discuss further in the next chapter on complexity, this formulation is particularly counterintuitive and causes scientists to hesitate to make declarative statements such as "Vaccines do not cause autism." Scientists are much more comfortable, simply because of the way experimentation is set up, to say something like "There is no difference in incidence of autism between vaccinated and non-vaccinated individuals." For most of us, this kind of statement is unsatisfactory because we are looking for the magic word *cause.* Yet, following Popper, scientific experimentation is not set up to establish *cause* but rather to disprove null hypotheses, and therefore a statement with the word *cause* is actually somewhat of a misrepresentation of the findings of scientific experimentation.

So why is it so difficult to establish a *cause* in a scientific experiment? As Popper observed, and as many modern scientists have lamented, it is because it is impossible to observe the very condition that would establish causality once and for all: the counterfactual. In 1973, David Lewis succinctly summarized the relationship between causality and the idea of the counterfactual:

> We think of a cause as something that makes a difference, and the difference it makes must be a difference from what would have

happened without it. Had it been absent, its effects—some of them, at least, and usually all—would have been absent as well.[1]

The counterfactual condition refers to what would have happened in a different world. For example, if I am trying to figure out whether drinking orange juice caused you to break out in hives, the precise way to determine this would be to go back in time and see what would have happened had you not had the orange juice. Everything would have been exactly the same, except for the consumption of orange juice. I could then compare the results of these two situations, and whatever differences I observe would have to be due to the consumption or non-consumption of orange juice, since this is the only difference in the two scenarios. You are the same you, you have the same exact experiences, and the environment you are in is exactly the same in both scenarios. The only difference is whether or not you drink the orange juice. This is the proper way to establish causality.

Since it is impossible to observe counterfactuals in real life (at least until we have developed the ability to go back in time), scientists often rely on randomized controlled trials to best approximate counterfactual effects. The thinking behind the randomized trial is that since everyone has an equal chance of being in either the control or experimental group, the people who get the treatment will not be systematically different from those randomized to get no treatment and therefore observed results can be attributed to the treatment. There are, however, many problems with this approach. Sometimes the two groups talk to each other and some of the experimental approach can even spill over into the control group, a phenomenon called "contamination" or "diffusion." Sometimes randomization does not work and the two groups turn out, purely by chance in most of these instances, to in fact be systematically different. Sometimes people drop out of the experiment in ways that make the two groups systematically different at the end of the experiment, a problem scientists refer to as "attrition bias."

Perhaps most important for epidemiological studies of the sort most relevant for the issues we deal with in this book, randomized controlled trials are often either impractical or downright unethical. For example, it would be impractical to randomly assign some people to eat GMOs and some people to not eat GMOs and then to see how many people in each group developed cancer. The development of cancer occurs slowly over many years, and it would be difficult to isolate the effects of GMOs versus all the other factors people are exposed to in their everyday lives that could contribute to cancer. Never mind the issue that a very substantial amount of the food we have been eating for the last decade in fact contains GMOs, making it a lot harder than might be thought to randomize people to a no-GMO group without their knowing it by virtue of the strange food they would be asked to eat. If we wanted to have a tightly controlled experiment to test this directly, we would have to keep people in both control and experimental groups quarantined in experimental quarters for most of their adult lives and control everything: from what they ate to what occupations they pursued to where they traveled. This would be costly, impractical, and, of course, unethical. We also could not randomize some severely depressed individuals to have ECT and others to no ECT, because if we believe that ECT is an effective treatment, it is unethical to deny the treatment to people who truly need it. In other words, once you have established the efficacy of a treatment, you cannot deny it to people simply for experimental purposes.

For all of these reasons, epidemiologists often rely on other experimental designs, including quasi-experimental designs, cohort studies, and case-control studies, many of which include following people with certain exposures and those without those exposures and seeing who develops particular diseases or conditions. The precise details of these different methods is less important for us now than what they have in common: instead of randomly assigning participants to different groups before starting the study, in these designs the research subjects have either already been or not been exposed to one or more conditions for reasons not under the researchers' control. Some people just happen to live near rivers that are polluted with industrial waste and others do not live as close to them; some people had the flu in 2009 and some didn't; some people drink a lot of green tea and others don't; or some people smoke and others don't.

In a world in which theories of causality ideally rely heavily on counterfactuals, these study designs are imperfect for a number of reasons. There are so many factors that determine why a person is in one of these groups, or *cohorts*, and not in the other that it is never an easy matter to isolate the most important ones. Take a study trying to find out if living near a polluted river increases the risk for a certain type of cancer. It could be that people who live near rivers own more boats and are exposed to toxic fumes from the fuel they use to power those boats or that more of them actually work at the factory that is polluting the river and are exposed to chemicals there that aren't even released into the river. If the researchers find more cancers in the group living near the polluted rivers, how do they know if the problem is the water pollution itself, inhaling fumes from boat fuel, or touching toxic chemicals in the factory?

On the other hand, cohort studies have managed to unearth findings as powerful as the irrefutable fact that cigarettes cause cancer. So while many of the tools we have at our disposal are imperfect, they are far from valueless. The problem is simply that establishing that cigarettes cause cancer required many decades of careful research and replicated studies before scientists were comfortable using the magic word "cause." The reluctance of scientists to use this word often has nothing to do with the strength of the evidence but is simply a remnant of the way scientists are taught to think about causality in terms of counterfactuals. Scientists will be reluctant to say the magic word until someone develops a time machine to allow us to observe actual counterfactual situations. In contrast, as Aristotle so astutely observed, laypeople are primed to look for causality in everything and to never feel secure until they have established it. This disconnect between the crude way in which we are all primed to think about causality and the ways in which scientists are trained to think about it causes a great deal of miscommunication and sometimes a sense of public distrust in scientists' knowledge.

Pies That Don't Satisfy

This brings us to a concept of causality used commonly in epidemiology that is for some reason very difficult to wrap our minds around: the sufficient-component cause model. Invented by epidemiologist Ken Rothman in 1976, this model is the subject of numerous multiple-choice questions for epidemiologists and public health students across the globe every year. As one of your authors with training in epidemiology knows, these are the questions that many students get wrong on the test. They are notoriously complex and sometimes even counterintuitive. The model imagines the causes of phenomena as a series of "causal pies." For example, *obesity* might be composed of several causal pies of different sorts. One pie might detail environmental causes, such as lack of a good walking environment, lack of healthy food options, and community or social norms. Another pie might include behavioral causes, such as a diet high in sugar and calories, lack of exercise, and a sedentary lifestyle. A third pie might include familial causes, such as poor parental modeling of healthy behaviors, a family culture of eating out or ordering takeout, and a lack of healthy food available in the home. A final pie might involve physiological factors like genes for obesity and hormonal abnormalities that cause obesity like Cushing's disease or hypothyroidism. Taken together, these different "pies" cause obesity in this model. For a cause to be necessary, it must occur in every causal pie. For example, if factor A needs to be present to cause Disease X, but other factors are also needed to cause Disease X, then the different pies will all have factor A in combination with other factors. If a cause is sufficient, it can constitute its own causal pie, even if there are other possible causes. For example, HIV is a sufficient cause of AIDS. HIV alone causes AIDS, regardless of what other factors are present.

In this model, causes can come in four varieties: necessary and sufficient, necessary but not sufficient, sufficient but not necessary, or neither sufficient nor necessary. The presence of a third copy of chromosome 21 is a necessary and sufficient cause of Down syndrome. Alcohol consumption is a necessary but not sufficient cause of alcoholism. In order to be classified as an alcoholic, alcohol consumption is necessary, but the fact of drinking alcohol in and of itself is not enough to cause alcoholism, or else everyone who drank alcohol would automatically be an alcoholic. Exposure to high doses of ionizing radiation is a sufficient but not necessary cause of sterility in men. This factor can cause sterility on its own but it is not the only cause of sterility, and sterility can certainly occur without it. A sedentary lifestyle is neither sufficient nor necessary to cause coronary heart disease. A sedentary lifestyle on its own will not cause heart disease, and heart disease can certainly occur in the absence of a sedentary lifestyle.

Although the model may seem abstract and overly complex, it is actually more relevant to everyday life and everyday health decisions than many people realize. For example, people who refuse to believe that cigarettes cause cancer (and there are still people who believe this, although there are many fewer than there were a few decades ago) often invoke the following refrain: "My aunt is 90 years old, smoked every day of her life, and she does not have lung cancer. Therefore, cigarettes cannot possibly cause lung cancer." This statement represents a misunderstanding of the sufficient-component cause model in its most devastating form. Smoking is neither a necessary nor sufficient cause of lung cancer. This means that lung cancer can develop in the absence of smoking and not everyone who smokes will develop lung cancer.[2] In other words, people who smoke may not develop lung cancer and people who do not smoke may develop lung cancer. But this does not mean that smoking is not *a* cause of lung cancer. It certainly is part of the causal pie. It just is not part of every causal pie and it cannot constitute its own causal pie, since the fact of smoking by itself does not produce lung cancer but must be accompanied by a personal genetic susceptibility to cigarette-induced mutations that cause cancer of the lungs. The model shows us that the fact that 90-year-old Aunt Ruth, who has been smoking two packs a day since 1935, does not have lung cancer is actually irrelevant. Smoking causes lung cancer, even if we do not observe cancer in every case of smoking. This is important, because, as we can see, a simple misunderstanding of the sufficient-component cause model can lead people to make incorrect assumptions about the health risks of certain behaviors.

As should be obvious by now, the concept of causality is a difficult one. Almost every intellectual you can think of, from philosophers to scientists, has probably pondered the definition of causality and how to establish it at some point. As we can see, there are a multitude of problems with inferring causality, and, in fact, many epidemiologists and research scientists would say that establishing causality is, in a sense, impossible. Since we cannot observe the counterfactual, we can never know for certain whether input A causes outcome B or whether they are simply strongly associated. Randomized controlled experiments are the closest we can come to a good approximation of the counterfactual condition, but they are often just not possible in our attempt to answer important questions about human health.

Cherry-Picking Yields Bad Fruit

Combine the healthy dose of skepticism with which professional scientists approach the establishment of causality with the natural human desire, noted by Aristotle, for causal mechanisms and we have a very real problem. Because causality is so difficult and because randomized controlled trials are only an approximation of the counterfactual condition, scientists must repeat experiments many times and observe the same result in order to feel some level of confidence in the existence of a causal relationship. Since the probability of finding the same results in numerous trials is relatively low if the true relationship has no causal valence, scientists can eventually begin to posit that a causal relationship exists. For example, the discovery that smoking cigarettes causes lung cancer did not occur overnight. Even though scientists had a strong hunch that this was the case, and there was certainly anecdotal evidence to support it, they had to wait until a number of carefully designed experiments with the appropriate statistical analyses could establish that the relationship was strong enough to be causal and that the observation of lung cancer following smoking was not simply due to random chance. Accompanied by the biological plausibility of nicotine's ability to cause carcinogenic mutations in lung cells, scientists were eventually able to communicate that the association between cigarette smoking and lung cancer was in all probability causal.

This point, about the necessity for multiple experimental demonstrations of the same effect before causality is declared, has another very important implication: in general, the results of a single experiment should not be taken as proof of anything. Unfortunately, the proselytes of anti-science ideas are constantly making this error. Thus, if 50 experiments contradict their beliefs and a single experiment seems consistent with them, certain individuals will seize upon that one experiment and broadcast it, complete with accusations that scientists knew about it all along but were covering up the truth. This is often referred to as *cherry-picking the data*.

While scientists verify and replicate the results of these experiments, we are always reluctant to wait patiently for an "answer." And this is exactly what Aristotle observed. People are not comfortable with observing phenomena in their environments that cannot be explained. As a result, they come up with their own explanations. In many instances, these explanations are incorrect, and, as we shall see, they are very often based on misinterpretations of coincidence. Here, the rational brain's ability to test and establish causality is completely at odds with the evolutionary impulse to assign causal explanations to everything in sight. The former requires long periods of thought, consideration, and a constant rethinking of what we even mean by *cause*. The latter feels necessary for everyday survival, to navigate a complex environment, and to satisfy a basic need to feel that the unknown is at least knowable.

Coincidence? I Think Not

A few months ago, one of us (Sara) lost the charger for her laptop and had to find a replacement. The replacement charger had an unusual feature: it needed a moment before the computer registered that the laptop was charging after being plugged in. Perhaps this was because this was not the charger originally designed for this particular laptop. In any case, the first time Sara plugged in her laptop with the new charger, she moved the laptop closer to the electrical socket and noticed that as she was doing this, the computer registered the charge. Sara immediately thought: "The laptop must need to be a certain distance from the electrical socket for the charger to work" and continued this ritual every time she plugged in her computer. One day, her husband interrupted her right after she plugged in her laptop and she did not have a chance to move the laptop closer to the electrical socket. When she sat back down at the computer, she saw that it had registered the charge. Being an adherent to the scientific method, Sara immediately realized that what she had thought to be a causal connection was a simple coincidence and that the real element that allowed the computer to register the charge was not the distance from the electrical socket but rather the simple passage of time. Nevertheless, the next time she plugged in her computer, she did not simply wait for the laptop to register the charge. Instead, she continued her ritual of moving the laptop closer to the electrical socket in what she rationally knew was a futile effort while she waited for the laptop to register the charge. Our readers will immediately recognize that this behavior has an element of confirmation bias to it: Sara refused to give up a belief she had acquired despite the presentation of new evidence to the contrary. But this time look at it from the perspective of causality. The new evidence specifically disconfirms the hypothesis that moving the computer closer to the electrical source causes the computer to register the charge.

This story is not simply meant to demonstrate the fallibility of your authors (although they readily admit they are indeed thus). It succinctly demonstrates the power of the human desire for causality, the extreme discomfort we all have with coincidence, and the devious ways in which our psychological processes, most of which are intuitive, can overcome, mute, and even sometimes obliterate our rational brains. Indeed, this kind of discomfort with coincidence, even when we know the true cause, has been established in a significant number of classic psychological studies, including experiments by the great B. F. Skinner. What is it about coincidence that makes us so uncomfortable? For one thing, we are primed to appreciate and recognize patterns in our environment.[3] If you flash a dot on and off against a wall with a laser pointer and then another one on and off within a tight time frame, people will register this as the motion of one dot rather than the flashing of two distinct dots.[4] In other words, people prefer sequences, and they will go to great lengths to rid their environments of randomness. Simple reinforcement studies, such as with Pavlov's famous dogs, have shown that it is very difficult for us to dissociate things that have for whatever reason become associated in our minds. If your phone rang while you were eating carrots yesterday and then it rang again today while you were again eating carrots, we can probably all agree that this is most likely a coincidence. There is no reason to believe that eating carrots could possibly cause the phone to ring. But we guarantee you that if this happened to you on several occasions, as ridiculous as it is, the thought would cross your mind that maybe the act of eating carrots causes your phone to ring. You will know it is not true, and you may even feel silly for thinking of it, but your mind will almost certainly register the thought. In reality, you might have a routine in which you eat carrots at a certain time that is also a time when many people are home from work and make phone calls. Maybe your carrot cravings are associated with the period after work and before dinner and this time is likely to be associated with a larger volume of people who could potentially be available to call you. This is an example of two unrelated events co-occurring because of the presence of some common third variable. This example may seem ridiculous, but the principle holds true: our desire to attribute causality is strong enough to override even our own conscious rationality.

We Love Our Patterns

As we've just established, human beings are primed to look for contiguity. We react to patterns in our environment above all.[5] This means that if two events just happen to occur together, we tend to assign a *pattern* to them that assumes that these events occur together regularly for a particular reason. Given our Aristotelian-defined inclination to assign causality to observed phenomena, we will likely begin to believe that not only do these events occur together regularly but they also occur together regularly because one causes the other. A *belief* is therefore the simple association the brain makes between two events when event B follows event A. The next time A occurs, our brains learn to expect B to follow. This is the most basic kind of belief formation: "I believe that eating carrots causes the phone to ring, since the last time I ate carrots the phone rang and now the next time eating carrots occurs, my brain will come to expect the phone to ring again."

Psychologists have often noted that this kind of pattern and belief formation probably provided our primitive ancestors with an important survival advantage. Since these ancestors had little means available to them to systematically separate causal connections from coincidence, they learned to pay attention to every observed association and to assume causality, just in case.[6] For example, if you were once chased and injured by an animal with orange and black stripes, you might soon associate the colors orange and black with danger. When you see orange and black in your environment subsequently, you will become anxious, your sympathetic nervous system will be activated, your psychological shortcut for "Orange and black cause danger" will be activated, and you will exhibit avoidant behavior—that is, you will run as fast as you can. This behavior might cause you to avoid orange-and-black objects that are not actually dangerous to you, but at the same time it will also help you to avoid tigers and any other orange-and-black objects that *are* dangerous to you, and you will therefore be much more likely to survive than someone who has not developed this pattern recognition. Thus in the absence of the ability to parse out causal from noncausal factors, it was evolutionarily beneficial for primitive human beings to err on the side of caution and assign causality to situations that *might* be dangerous or to elements of clearly dangerous situations that may or may not be truly causal. This evolutionary benefit of over-assigning causality probably became hardwired in human brains and has now become a fact of everyday existence and a natural human inclination.

Stuck in a Pattern Jam

It would therefore not be an exaggeration to assert that we are most comfortable when we are aware of what causes the phenomena in our environments. We can think back to the last time we were stuck in a horrendous traffic jam. After cursing our luck and swearing a bit, our first thought was "Why? Why is there a traffic jam? Is it an accident? Rush hour? Construction? Is everyone just going to the Jersey Shore because it is a nice day? Is it a holiday?" Then we turned on the radio and tuned into the traffic channel, waiting anxiously for news about the traffic on our route. We did not pay much attention to traffic reports for the route before we set out, which might actually have been helpful since we might have been able to plan an alternative route. But once in the traffic jam, we became completely focused on hearing about why we were stuck in this particular traffic jam at this particular moment.

In reality, when you are sitting in the middle of a traffic jam that extends for many miles, listening to the traffic report and even knowing the cause of the traffic has no practical value. You cannot change your route because you are stuck, and the next exit is many miles away. You cannot get out of your car and take the subway or walk instead. You cannot go back in time and take an alternative route or rush to the scene of the accident, get the site cleared up, and fix the traffic problem more efficiently. There is literally nothing you can do about the situation you are in, and knowing its cause will do nothing to help you. Nevertheless, we feel a strong need to *know why*. We are not satisfied just waiting in the traffic, listening to some music, and eventually getting home. The comforting feeling of being able to assign causes to observed phenomena in our environments probably has a lot to do with the evolutionary advantage of recognizing patterns and causes discussed earlier. Since we are hardwired to look for causes and since recognizing causes once allowed us a significant evolutionary advantage, we will most often feel a great sense of relief when we figure out the cause of something. Knowing what caused the traffic jam didn't make it go away, but it did help us cope with it.

This is the sort of thinking that drives us to the doctor when we have unexplained symptoms. First and foremost, we believe that the doctor can offer us tangible relief and possibly even a cure. At the same time, we also take great relief in a diagnosis, not simply because it often moves us closer to a cure, but also because we intuitively feel better when we know the *why* behind the phenomena around us. How unsatisfied and even angry we feel if the doctor tells us she cannot find what is causing our symptoms, which is in fact very often the case. Unfortunately, this mentality leads both doctors and patients to embark on diagnostic test adventures. Our healthcare system is being bankrupted by unnecessary MRIs, CAT scans, and other expensive tests in futile searches for a *cause* that will make us feel we are in control. In medical school doctors are taught: "Do not order a test unless you know that the result of that test will make a difference in the treatment you recommend to the patient." Yet, confronted with a patient who has symptoms, that wisdom goes right out the window. A doctor may know very well that the best treatment for a patient complaining of back pain who has a normal neurological examination is exercise and physical therapy. In the great majority of cases, nothing that turns up on an MRI of the back, even a herniated disc, will change that approach. But doctors still order the MRI so that they can tell the patient "Your back pain is caused by a herniated disc."[7] Then the doctor recommends exercise and physical therapy.

We therefore create a world of "arbitrary coherence," as Dan Ariely has termed it.[8] Our existence as "causal-seeking animals"[9] means that the kinds of associations and correlations that researchers notice in the process of attempting to establish causality are immediately translated into true and established causes in our minds. We can know rationally that association does not prove causation, and we can even recognize examples in which this kind of thinking is a fallacy, and all the same, our innate psychological processes will still undermine us and assign causality whenever possible. And as many researchers have established, once we come to believe something, once we formulate our hypothesis that carrot-eating causes phone-ringing, we are extremely slow to change our beliefs, even if they have just been formulated or have been formulated on the basis of weak or inconsistent evidence.[10]

What does all of this mean for our evaluation of health-related information? Many phenomena associated with health are actually coincidental. For example, it is possible to have an allergic rash in re-action to a medication and also have an upset stomach, but the two symptoms might be coincidental rather than related. This is actually quite common in everyday life, but we tend to believe that any symp-toms we have at the same time must be all causally related to the same condition.

It Really Is Just a Coincidence

In terms of health topics discussed in this book, coincidence can be interpreted as causality when no clear cause has been identified by science. The most potent example is the vaccines-autism issue. Scientists have some ideas about factors that may contribute to autism, such as older age of the father at conception and certain risk genes, but for the most part, the causes are a mystery.[11] It becomes even more difficult to conceptualize cause in the case of chronic diseases, for which contributing factors can be diverse and every individual can have a different combination of risk factors that cause the same disease. The timing of childhood vaccines and of the onset of autism are so close that they can be considered synchronous. This synchronicity opens up the potential for coinci-dence to be interpreted as cause. Indeed, many people have viewed the rise in rates of autism and the synchronous rise in volume of childhood vaccines as more than coincidence. They insist that adding vaccines to the childhood regimen "overwhelms" the child's immune system and results in devastating chronic health outcomes, including autism.

A similar coincidence could be observed with nuclear power and cancer. A rise in cases of cancer in a particular town might coin-cide in time with the building of a nuclear power plant. Based on what we know about the development of cancer, it is very unlikely that a nuclear power plant could immediately cause cancer. Even if there were an association between nuclear power plants and cancer, it would take a long time for cancer cases to rise after the building of the plant. But our innate search for causality might cause us to view this coincidence as cause and immediately decide that even the building of a nuclear power plant is a real cause of devastating disease.

The interpretation of coincidence as cause is extremely common in misunderstandings of disease causality and health dangers, and, as we have seen, the complexity of establishing cause in medical science and the divergence between the ways scientists and the rest of us conceptualize cause exacerbates the situation further, as we discussed in the introduction.

Rabbit Feet and Other Strange Beliefs

Many definitions of *superstition* involve the notion that superstition is established by a false assignment of cause and effect.[12] Superstition is an extremely powerful human inclination that perfectly fits the notion of filling the ignorance gap. We cannot know why many things around us happen, so we invent reasons or ways to try to control occurrences and we assign causes to nonrelated incidents that may have occurred alongside an event. We all know how this works, of course, and we are all guilty of engaging in superstition, even if we do not consider ourselves particularly superstitious people. We might re-wear clothing that we thought brought us good luck at a recent successful interview or eat the same cereal before a test that we ate before another test on which we performed well. These are examples of superstitious behavior. Many psychologists, medical researchers, and philosophers have framed superstition as a cognitive error. Yet in his 1998 book *Why People Believe Weird Things: Pseudoscience, Superstition, and Other Confusions of Our Time*, Michael Shermer challenges the notion that superstition is altogether irrational. Shermer effectively asks why superstition would be so pervasive if it were a completely irrational, harmful behavior. Shermer hypothesizes that in making causal associations, humans confront the option to deal with one of two types of errors that are described in classic statistical texts: Type I errors involve accepting something that is not true, and Type II errors involve rejecting something that is true. Shermer proposes that in situations in which committing a Type II error would be detrimental to survival, natural selection favors strategies that involve committing Type I errors. Hence superstitions and false beliefs about cause and effect arise.[13] This is precisely the argument we made earlier with our example about avoiding orange and black after an attack by an orange-and-black animal: erring on the side of caution and believing something that may not be true is more beneficial than potentially rejecting something that may be true—for example, that everything orange and black is a threat.

We Are All Pigeons

How do we know that superstitious beliefs are so pervasive? Many of us consider ourselves rational and might reject the notion that we have superstitious inclinations. Yet classic experiments by some of the greatest psychologists, including B. F. Skinner, have demonstrated how natural and ubiquitous superstitious behavior is, even among nonhuman species. Skinner's experiments on superstitious behaviors in pigeons have become some of the most powerful evidence in favor of the idea that superstition is a natural, almost automatic, response in a variety of species. In one experiment, Skinner placed a hungry pigeon in a chamber where a feeder automatically released food every 15 seconds. At first, the pigeon was stationary and waited for the food every 15 seconds. After some time had passed, however, each pigeon developed distinctive rituals while waiting for the food to be released. Some walked in circles, some engaged in head thrusting, and others bobbed their heads.[14] The interesting finding here is that even though the pigeons had already learned that the food was released automatically every 15 seconds, they still developed rituals while they were waiting that were continuously reinforced by the automatic release of the food after 15 seconds. Once the rituals were reinforced by the release of the food, they were simply strengthened in the minds of the pigeons, who then continued these particular rituals without fail until the end of the experiment. This experiment suggests that animals have some form of innate desire for control over causation. An unknown cause, such as an unknown mechanism releasing food every 15 seconds, is not acceptable. This example is exactly like Sara's ritual of moving the computer closer to the electric socket, even though she had already learned that time was the real cause of the computer's registering of the charge. Either Sara has the mind of a pigeon, or this need to fill the causal ignorance gap is so strong and so basic that all species, from pigeons to dogs to monkeys to humans, are capable of engaging in superstitious rituals to establish control over the outcomes observed in their environments.

A similar experiment with children established the same point. In this experiment, children ages 3 to 6 first chose a toy they wanted, then they were introduced to Bobo, a clown doll who automatically dispensed marbles every 15 seconds. If enough marbles gathered, the child would get the toy. Even though the children knew that Bobo automatically dispensed marbles every 15 seconds, they still developed unique ritual behaviors. Some children started touching Bobo's nose, some smiled at Bobo, others grimaced at him. This experiment again showed that people want to create causes they have control over and they want to be able to explain effects through their own actions.[16]

According to a Gallup poll, about 50% of Americans believe that some kind of superstitious behavior, such as rubbing a rabbit's foot, will result in a positive outcome, such as doing well on a test.[15] Superstitious behaviors and beliefs may be reinforced because they seem to improve people's performance. In one experiment, college students were given 10 attempts to putt a golf ball. Students who were told that the ball was "lucky" performed significantly better than those who were told nothing. Similarly, students who were given a task to perform in the presence of a "lucky charm" performed significantly better than students with no "lucky charms."[17] These types of experiments show us not only that superstition can be reinforced but also that, once again, irrational beliefs may be beneficial to us in some way. After all, superstition did improve the students' performances without any negative consequences. As we have discussed throughout this book, being strictly rational is not always the most immediately adaptive strategy. Unfortunately, however, eschewing reason can produce disastrous misconceptions in situations in which rational objectivity is truly needed.

The Dreaded 2 × 2 Table

What are some of the fallacies, other than superstition and disbelief in coincidence, that people make when it comes to cause and effect? One major source of misunderstanding of cause and effect is our general inability to understand independent events. We tend to think that the probability of one event depends on the probability of another. If I just sat in traffic passing through Connecticut on my way to New York from Boston, I may conjecture that one traffic jam per trip is enough and that I am unlikely to hit traffic in New York. This is incorrect, because the probability of traffic in Connecticut and the probability of traffic in New York are independent phenomena that may or may not be influenced by a common third factor, like the fact that it is a holiday and many people are therefore on the road. Experiencing traffic in Connecticut does nothing to affect the probability of experiencing traffic in New York because the events are independent, even though you are experiencing them continuously. This is the central concept behind the *gambler's fallacy*. People tend to think that the world is somehow "even," so that if we spin 25 blacks in a row on the roulette wheel, we feel certain that the next spin has to be red. In reality, each spin is independent, and the fact of spinning 25 blacks in a row does not affect the probability of a red on the next spin.[18]

Why do we make these mistakes? Cognitive psychologists have found that we are susceptible to two types of bias that make us more likely to make these particular kinds of errors. The first is the illusory correlation, a bias that leads us to believe that things are related when they are not and describes things like Sara's belief about her computer charger. The second is an attentional bias, in which we pay too much attention to certain types of information and not others. To illustrate how this one works, it is best to think about a standard 2 × 2 table, a favorite of biostatisticians and epidemiologists, often to the dismay of their students. Table 2 is a classic example of a 2 × 2 table that epidemiologists and statisticians would use.

This is a sight that will send shudders down the backs of everyone who has ever taken a biostatistics course, and understandably so. The presentation of data in this way and the thinking that goes along with it is not intuitive. That is why when students see a table

TABLE 2 A Classic 2 × 2 Table

	Lung Cancer	No Lung Cancer	Total
Smoked cigarettes	95	55	150
Did not smoke cigarettes	5	145	150
Total	100	200	300

like this, they have to think about it for a while, they have to check any calculations they do with the table extensively, and they have to make sure they understand what the table is getting at before making any assumptions about the relationship between the exposure and the disease. So, what does this table mean, and how would we use it?

The table represents a complete picture of the relationship between exposure to cigarettes and the development of lung cancer. By *complete*, we do not mean that it captures the entire population, because obviously these numbers indicate only a sample of the population and capturing the entire population is always close to impossible. We use this term simply to indicate that the 2 × 2 table allows us to think about *all* of the possibilities associated with the exposure. The table allows us to think not only about the people who smoke cigarettes and develop cancer, but also about those who smoke cigarettes and do not develop cancer. It also allows us to think not only about those who do not smoke and do not develop cancer, but also about those who do not smoke and do develop cancer. The attentional bias effectively means that our inclination in these types of situations is to focus only on the first number, 95, in the upper left-hand corner of the 2 × 2 table, and not on the other numbers.[19] Inventive studies with nurses and patient records have even confirmed this way of thinking among healthcare professionals.[20] This means that we are always looking for a causal association, such as "Cigarette smoking causes lung cancer," without first examining the entire picture. Now, of course, we do know that cigarette smoking causes cancer. But what if instead of smoking and cancer, we had put "vaccines" and "autism"? If you looked only at the upper left-hand corner, you would of course see some number of people who had a vaccine and had autism. But looking at the whole table, you should see why assuming therefore that vaccines cause, or are even associated with, autism based on just the upper left-hand corner would be a huge mistake. This number needs to be compared with the number of children who are not vaccinated who have autism and with the number of children who are vaccinated and do not have autism. On its own, the number of children with both vaccinations and autism is meaningless. But the attentional bias is a cognitive heuristic we use all the time to ignore the other parts of the 2 × 2 table.

So the next time someone asserts an association between a potential exposure and disease, see if you can draw out the corresponding

2 × 2 table and then ask them to fill in the blanks. Using your 2 × 2 table, you can ask questions like "You say you found that 150 people who lived near a nuclear power plant developed cancer. How many people developed cancer in a similar area without a nuclear power plant?" You would be surprised at how often the rest of the table is neglected. Now you have learned how to help fill it in.

So What Should We Do About It?

Now that we have delineated all of the ways in which our minds try to fill in the ignorance gap by promoting causes for effects that may not be truly related, we have to figure out some strategies for avoiding these kinds of mental traps. We already outlined a few, including constructing a 2 × 2 table and asking yourself, "What is in the other boxes in this scenario?" We have hopefully also made you more aware of the ways in which our minds immediately jump to causes when we are sitting in a traffic jam or have a headache and a stomachache at the same time ("There must be a common cause," our minds immediately trick us into thinking). In addition, we have talked a bit about independent events and demonstrated that the probability of one independent event happening has nothing to do with the probability of the occurrence of another independent event.

In addition to these strategies of avoiding the trap of the causal ignorance gap, we would like to include some recommendations for ways in which we can be more aware of how we think about causes and strategies to help prevent us from jumping to conclusions. One suggestion involves teaching children about cause and effect at a young age. This would include not only teaching them what causes and effects are, but also, at a more advanced grade level, training them to be skeptical of easy causal answers and teaching them more about the history of various definitions of causality. Some school curricula, most notably the Common Core, already embrace this topic. Figure 3 shows an example of a cause-and-effect worksheet for second graders from the Common Core.

These kinds of worksheets help young children think logically about cause and effect and can be very helpful in embedding the concept at a young age. Curriculum materials for older children could include assignments that involve finding an existing causal claim, perhaps on the Internet, and writing a short paper about whether

Name: _____

Cause & Effect

Read the cause and write an effect. Then, write one full sentence that states the cause and effect.

example: **Cause:** A blizzard hit the city.

        Effect: *All the schools were closed.*

        Sentence: *A blizzard hit the city, so all the schools were closed.*

1.   **Cause:** I planted some sunflower seeds.

    Effect: _____

    Sentence: _____

2.   **Cause:** My sister stayed up past midnight.

    Effect: _____

    Sentence: _____

3.   **Cause:** Lizzy spilled milk all over the floor.

    Effect: _____

    Sentence: _____

4.   **Cause:** David signed up for guitar lessons.

    Effect: _____

    Sentence: _____

FIGURE 3 Cause and effect worksheet.

Source: From http://www.superteacherworksheets.com/causeeffectfactopinion/causeeffect2_WBMBD.pdf

or not the claim is defensible, how sound the evidence is for it, how logical it is, and what some other causes could be. Extending some of the specialized critical thinking skills that students of epidemiology gain at a graduate level could be extremely valuable for the general population. These kinds of skills include the ability to assess study designs for bias, the ability to think through the validity of causal claims, and the ability to identify competing biases and alternative explanations for phenomena that seem causally related. Many of the curriculum materials on these subjects for high school students could simply be extracted from epidemiology syllabi and simplified for a broader view of thinking critically about causality. These sorts of exercises will benefit a student no matter what field he or she ultimately chooses, because learning how to think in a systematic and logical manner about the phenomena we see in the world around us and learning how to articulate an argument in support of or in opposition to existing claims about our environments are highly transferable skills. They simply represent the core of critical thinking abilities that are in demand in every sector of the workplace and are essential to success in higher education and beyond.

Of course, if you are conversing with someone who is completely convinced by an unscientific claim like vaccines cause autism or guns are good protection, you are unlikely to have much of an effect on him or her. However, a lot of the advice in this book is geared toward getting the very large number of people who are "on the fence" to accept the proven scientific evidence rather than the emotional arguments of the Jenny McCarthys of the world. If you find yourself speaking with a young parent who is afraid of getting his or her children vaccinated because of what he or she has heard about the potential "dangers" of vaccines, you can actually use a variety of techniques outlined in this chapter and in other places in the book to help guide your acquaintance to the evidence. We will discuss motivational interviewing as a technique that helps people face and resolve ambivalence at greater length in chapter 5.

Motivate the Inner Scientist

In the case of a conversation with a young parent who is reluctant to vaccinate his or her child, you can try motivational interviewing techniques yourself as part of a normal dialogue. In order for these techniques to be successful, you need to express empathy, support the person's self-efficacy (that is, her ability to believe that she has power over the events in her life and the decisions she makes and the capacity to change her opinion about something), and to be able to tolerate the person's resistance to what you are saying. You need to ask open-ended questions and to be able to draw out your conversation companion. For example, if this person tells you that she thinks vaccines are dangerous and she is thinking of not getting her children vaccinated, the best first thing to say to this statement is not "That is not true—there is no evidence that vaccines are dangerous," but rather to gently prod the person into exploring her feelings further by saying something to the effect of "Tell me more" or "How did you come to feel nervous about vaccines?" You can then guide the person through a slowed-down, articulated version of her thought process in getting to the conclusion "Vaccines are dangerous," and along the way you can get her to express her main desire, to keep her children healthy. This technique can help people begin to feel more comfortable with their ambivalence, slow down and think more carefully and calmly about an important decision such as whether or not to get their children vaccinated, and guide them toward more intelligent questions about the issue and a better understanding of their own fears and concerns. Of course, this technique will not always work and it may take more than one encounter with a person to really have an impact, but it is always better to err on the side of empathy and reflective listening rather than showering the person with all the facts that oppose her point of view. Most of us already know that the latter strategy pretty much never works.

Another tactic you can take is simply to help the person see the whole 2 × 2 table rather than just the upper left-hand corner. Again, you have to be gentle and not simply throw facts at the person to prove her "wrong." Instead, you should show interest in her opinion and then simply ask her to elaborate: "That's interesting. Do you know how many children who are vaccinated are diagnosed with autism within the year?" And then you can start asking the difficult questions: "I wonder how many children who are not vaccinated get autism." By asking some of these questions, you may trigger a wider awareness in the person and help guide her toward a fuller understanding of how causality is determined in science, especially in epidemiology. However, if you simply tell her that she does not understand the true nature of causality and that she needs to study 2 × 2 tables, you will do nothing but alienate her and make her even less likely to examine her ambivalence and the foundations of her ideas.

Making causal inferences is absolutely necessary in negotiating our daily lives. If I am driving and start to doze off at the wheel, I am going to assume that insomnia the previous night is the cause of the problem and pull over and take a nap lest I cause an accident. We are required to do this all the time, and sometimes we even have fun with it: many of us love to be entertained by detective shows in which "Who did it?" is really asking the question of causality. But when making critical decisions about health and healthcare for ourselves and our families, we need to be extremely careful and understand how naturally prone we are to leap to conclusions. Scientists and doctors fall into the trap as well. Since we are all guilty of misplaced causal theories, it is critical that we help each other fill in the rest of those boxes.

Avoidance of Complexity

E VERY DAY SCORES OF SCIENTIFIC ARTICLES ARE PUBLISHED THAT report on the results of studies examining the causes and treatments of diseases. Each of these articles usually has five sections:

1. *Abstract:* an overall summary of what the paper is about
2. *Introduction:* an explanation of what the problem is and why the present study may offer new insights
3. *Methods:* a detailed account of exactly what the investigators did, usually including a statistical section in which the authors explain what mathematical tools they used to decide if their results are meaningful
4. *Results:* the data collected during the study (full of numbers, tables, and figures)
5. *Discussion:* the conclusion, in which the scientists explain the significance of their findings, what shortcomings their study had, and what should be done next to further understanding of the field in question

It is hoped that other biomedical scientists and clinicians will read as many of these papers as possible so that they can keep up-to-date on the newest information. We expect that our doctors are on the cutting edge of medical science. But of course no individual can approach reading all of these papers, even if he or she narrows the field down by reading only the most relevant topics. Furthermore, scientific papers generally do not make the most gripping reading. Although editors of scientific journals expect the papers they publish to conform to proper spelling, grammar, and syntax, they place a premium on conveying scientific accuracy, not on producing page-turners. So at the end of a long day in the laboratory or clinic, what parts of a paper do scientists and clinicians actually read?

The first thing to be ignored is the Methods section. A typical Methods section is full of technical details about who or what the subjects of the study were, what measurements were made, how the data were collected and stored, how informed consent was obtained if human subjects were involved, and what kinds of statistical analyses were done. Of course, this is the most important part of the paper. A careful reading of the Methods section in a paper published in even the most reputable and prestigious journals—such as *Science, Nature,* and the *New England Journal of Medicine*—almost never fails to reveal at least one thing that could be questioned, or one assumption or compromise that the investigators had to make in order to get the study done. But the Methods section just seems so "complicated," and it is easiest to assume that the reviewers of the paper and the editors of the journal have made sure everything was done properly. Why not just look at the abstract, see what was found out, and leave it at that?

Scientists often throw up their hands at what they perceive to be the lack of "scientific literacy" on the part of the "general public" (e.g., nonscientists). Articles are published every year detailing some study that seems to show that Americans are scientifically less adept than residents of other developed countries. Most people take the easy way out, the scientists lament, and prefer believing superficial, often incorrect, descriptions of scientific knowledge and findings to delving into the truth. There is no doubt that these assertions are at least to some degree correct, and we will return to them later in this chapter. But as we described in the beginning of this chapter, even scientists are prone to reach for the easiest available method of getting information. It is only human nature to avoid complexity whenever possible in order to get information about a complicated topic.

Science is not necessarily the most complicated field we deal with, even if scientists sometimes want us to believe that to be the case. The most brilliant scientist may have a great deal of trouble understanding the details of the annual changes to federal accounting regulations, the rules of evidence regarding criminal procedure, or just exactly what is going on in James Joyce's novel *Finnegan's Wake*. Those things require appropriate experts, an accountant, a lawyer, and an English literature professor. But no one disputes that modern science involves challenging complexities that seem well beyond the grasp of even the most intelligent nonspecialist. And every area of science, including those within the medical and health fields with which we are concerned in this book, has its own set of complexities, including jargon, standards, and abbreviations. This chapter details another human impulse—avoidance of complexity—that is so natural to us for a variety of beneficial reasons but also causes an enormous amount of false belief when it comes to rational scientific thinking. We begin by looking at how the quest for simplicity affects us all, even the most seasoned of scientists; detail some of the ways in which our brains are primed to misunderstand science and eschew rationality; and finally propose some possible methods to make scientific thinking more intuitive. We also provide some simplified frameworks to help people break down seemingly complex scientific information into more manageable and interpretable issues. Finally, we offer suggestions about how to tell which science websites are giving us accurate information.

Science Illiteracy Has Multiple Culprits

It does not help matters when a tabloid newspaper, the *New York Daily News*, laments our general lack of scientific sophistication with the banner headline "Idiocracy: Much of U.S. Doesn't Buy Big Bang or Evolution."[1] The story tells us that according to a "new poll" conducted by the Associated Press, 51% of people don't think the Big Bang happened and 40% don't believe in evolution. The story goes on to make fun of the average citizen who questions the Big Bang "theory" because "I wasn't there."

The problems with this kind of media sensationalism are manifold. First, not a single detail about the poll from which the story derives is given, so we have no idea whether it is valid. A scientist or an informed consumer of science should ask "Who was surveyed, what was the 'return rate' (the number of people approached who agreed to be surveyed), and what does the statistical analysis of the data tell us about whether any firm conclusions can actually be reached?" Second, buried at the end of the story is the good news: only 4% of people doubt that smoking cigarettes causes cancer, only 6% question whether mental illness is a medical condition, and only 8% disagree that our cells carry the genetic code.

But finally, and most important, is the attack on the average American, who is being labeled an "idiot." We do not need sophisticated psychological experiments to tell us that epithets like that are unlikely to motivate anyone to want to learn more about the Big Bang or about evolution. And it also discourages scientists, doctors, and public health officials from trying to teach them. The article could have started with the remarkable information that a concerted public health campaign has convinced almost everyone that smoking is dangerous, despite the influence of the tobacco industry, or that even though the discovery of the structure of the genetic molecule, DNA, was published only in 1953 it is already the case that nearly everyone agrees that our genes determine what our bodies do and look like. Clearly, we need to do more work to help people understand that the Big Bang and evolution are real and indisputable phenomena and that even religious people for the most part agree with that fact. But calling people "idiots" is a setback. In addition, it takes our attention away from the real question: If people can understand science in many instances, why do they deny health and medical facts in some cases and not others? Saying it is because they are "uneducated" is, in this sense, the easy way out.

Indeed, the media can sometimes be a culprit in fostering scientific misunderstandings and myths. In a penetrating op-ed piece, Frank Bruni of *The New York Times* wonders why a former Playboy model, Jenny McCarthy, was able to gain so much attention with the notion that vaccines cause autism. He asks, "When did it become O.K. to present gut feelings like hers as something in legitimate competition with real science? That's what the interviewers who gave her airtime did ... and I'd love to know how they justify it."[2] The media will always claim that they present only what people want to hear, and it is undoubtedly more pleasurable for many people to watch Jenny McCarthy being interviewed than to listen to a scientist drone on and on about the immunological basis of vaccination. How, then, will people learn about scientific truths? Rather than brand us as idiots, the media might try a little harder to educate us about science.

We Are Not Stupid

It is important to recognize that the issue here is not one of intelligence. It is all too often the case that scientists, physicians, and public health authorities assume that anyone who fails to agree with the conclusions reached by scientific inquiry must be simply stupid. In accord with that viewpoint, educational interventions are developed that seem overly simplistic or even condescending. But the retreat from complexity and the unwillingness to plumb the depths of scientific detail afflicts even the smartest among us.

We cannot, however, lay the blame for fear of scientific complexity and pandering to the simplest explanations solely at the feet of the media, for the scientific community bears a great deal of responsibility as well. In 2013 Dan M. Kahan traced the way Americans were informed about the approval and introduction of a new vaccine against the human papillomavirus (HPV), the sexually transmitted virus that is the cause of cervical cancer.[3] When the vaccine was introduced by the drug company Merck under the brand name Gardasil in 2006 it was accompanied by a CDC recommendation for universal immunization of adolescent girls and a campaign by the drug company to get state legislatures to mandate Gardasil immunization. The result was enormous controversy, with anti-vaxxers insisting the vaccine had been rushed to approval and other groups raising the concern that the vaccine would somehow encourage adolescents to have sex.[4] What struck Kahan about this is the fact that the hepatitis B (another sexually transmitted virus that causes cancer) vaccine, which was introduced in the 1990s, did not evoke anywhere near the public outcry or controversy and is now an accepted part of the routine vaccination schedule for children. The difference, Kahan contends, is the way in which the scientific and regulatory communities handled the introduction of Gardasil to the public. "There was and remains no process in the FDA or the CDC for making evidence-based assessment of the potential impact of their procedures on the myriad everyday channels through which the public becomes apprised of decision-relevant science," Kahan wrote. First, the FDA fast-tracked approval of Gardasil, allowing Merck to get a leg up on its competitor, GlaxoSmithKline's Cervarix. Then, Merck went about a very public lobbying campaign. Finally, the CDC recommended vaccinating girls but not boys. These decisions managed to push every button in everyone's arsenal of fear and mistrust. Rather than hearing about Gardasil from their pediatricians, as they had with the hepatitis B vaccine, parents first learned about it in sensationalized media accounts. Kahan puts the blame squarely on the FDA, CDC, Merck, and the medical community for not even considering how Americans would interpret their decisions:

> Empirically, uniformed [sic] and counterproductive risk communication is the inevitable by-product of the absence of a systematic, evidence-based alternative. . . . The failure of democratic societies to use scientific knowledge to protect the science communication environment from influences that prevent citizens from recognizing that decision-relevant science contributes to their well-being.

Complicated Science Confounds the Brightest Among Us

Let us suppose that a parent with a PhD in history, Dr. Smith, is trying to decide whether to have his children vaccinated for measles, mumps, and rubella. He understands that these potentially very serious and even fatal diseases have nearly disappeared from the population because of vaccines. He is a generally civic-minded person who under ordinary circumstances has no problem doing what is best for other people in his community. But his paramount interest is the welfare and health of his own children, a priority few of us would dispute. He has heard that children are exposed to so many vaccinations at such an early age that the immune system is overtaxed and ultimately weakened. Children who undergo the full set of vaccinations supposedly are at high risk to succumb later in life to a variety of immunological diseases—including food allergies, behavioral problems, and seizures—because of vaccines. He has seen data that rates of these illnesses are increasing in the American population and that these increases have occurred in lock step with the proliferation of vaccinations. We cannot blame our history professor for being concerned that by vaccinating his children he may ultimately be responsible for harming them.

So the dutiful, loving parent decides to learn more about vaccines. Perhaps he goes online first, but he quickly realizes this is a mistake. There are articles on all sides of the issue, many written by people with impressive sounding scientific credentials (lots of MDs and PhDs and award-winning scientists from prestigious colleges and universities). He decides to focus on information provided by medical societies of pediatrics and immunology. What does he find out?

Some viruses and bacteria are immediately cleared from the body by a part of the immune system called the innate immune system, which includes natural killer cells, macrophages, and dendritic cells. These are not stimulated by vaccinations. Instead, it is another part of the immune system, the adaptive immune system, that responds to vaccinations. The adaptive immune system is in turn comprised of the humoral and cell-mediated immune systems, the former mediated by B cells, which produce antibodies and the latter by T cells, which are often called CD cells and have designations like "CD4+ and CD8+." Antibodies include a light fragment and a heavy fragment . . .

We could go on with this, but hopefully we have made our point. Although our history professor would have no trouble delving into the effects of a new form of taxation on relations between the aristocratic and middle classes in 14th-century Flanders, when researching how a vaccine might affect his child he is already lost in the whirlwind of letters, abbreviations, and arrows from one type of immune cell to the next. And what we have provided above is merely scratching the surface. The human immune system is one of the most beautifully organized systems in the universe, capable of protecting us against the barrage of dangerous microbes we face every second of our lives. But those microbes are also brilliant in their ability to elude and co-opt the immune system in order to cause disease. How vaccines fit into this system, which has developed over millions of years of evolution to make the human species so capable of long-term survival, is ultimately a very complicated affair.

After a few hours of trying to understand the science behind immunization, Dr. Smith decides to settle on something simpler. He can easily find much briefer summaries of how vaccines work on the

Internet. Most of these seem to him to be too simple, some even to the point of feeling condescending. They represent many points of view, some insisting that vaccines are safe and others that they are nearly poisonous. Dr. Smith is now getting tired and knows that at some point he will have to make a decision. Instead of trying to weed through all the technical details of the scientific reports, he decides to go with a vividly designed website sponsored by an organization called the National Association for Child and Adolescent Immunization Safety (a fictitious organization), presided over by the fictitious Ronald Benjamin Druschewski, PhD, MD, RN, MSW, MBA, ABCD (again, we are being deliberately hyperbolic here to emphasize our point). The site makes the case simply and forcefully that vaccinations stress the child's immune system, that "long-term studies have not been done to evaluate the safety of multiple vaccinations" and that "studies show that many children are harmed every day by immunizations." The site proceeds to give the gripping story of one 5-year-old boy who is now plagued with allergies to multiple food types and can safely eat only a pureed diet of mashed carrots and sweet potatoes without developing wheezing and hives.

Dr. Smith decides not to vaccinate his children and to turn in for the night.

The situation just outlined illustrates many different factors that cause science denial, but we emphasize here just one of them: the *avoidance of complexity*. Despite the fact that he is a superbly well educated and intelligent person, Dr. Smith is not an immunologist and yet he is faced with tackling either very technical discussions of the biological basis for immunization or overly simplified ones. Despite making an honest effort, he is ultimately defeated by complexity, believes he will never be able to understand the issues with any sort of rigor, and defaults to explanations that are much easier to grasp albeit less accurate.

Most people do not have PhDs and do not have as high an IQ as Dr. Smith, but people of average intelligence and educational background will also face the same dilemma if they attempt to understand the scientific basis behind many facets of medical advice. It is not easy to understand how a gene can be inserted into the genome of a plant in order to render it resistant to droughts or insects. Nor are the data demonstrating that keeping a gun at home is dangerous straightforward for someone who wishes to understand them in depth: such data are derived from epidemiological studies that require complicated statistical analyses. Even many of the people who perform such studies need to collaborate with expert statisticians in order to get the math right. Once an equation shows up, most people—even very intelligent people—get nervous.

Dealing With Complexity Requires Considerable Mental Energy

Neuroscientists, cognitive psychologists, and behavioral economists have developed a theory in recent years that divides mental processes into two varieties, variously referred to as the high road versus the low road, system 1 versus system 2, the reflective system versus the reflexive system, or fast thinking versus slow thinking. We have stressed that this dichotomy is a serious oversimplification of how the mind works. Nevertheless, it is very clear from abundant research that humans have retained more primitive parts of the brain, present in all mammals, which are used to make rapid, emotional decisions. As the great neuroscientist Joseph LeDoux of New York University has shown, one key part of the emotional brain is the amygdala, an almond-shaped structure deep in what is called the limbic cortex of the mammalian brain.[5] On the other hand, humans are unique in the size and sophistication of the portion of the brain to which we have referred on a number of occasions so far, the prefrontal cortex, or PFC, which we use to perform logical operations based on reason and reflection. Almost all parts of the human brain, including the amygdala and its related structures in the limbic cortex, are barely distinguishable from those of other mammals, including our nearest genetic neighbor, the chimpanzee. The PFC, shown in figure 4, however, is the part of the brain that makes us uniquely human, for better (writing novels and composing symphonies) or worse (waging war and insider trading). Again, the tendency on the part of some authors to talk about the PFC as the seat of reason is a vast oversimplification of a brain region that contains billions of neurons, multiple layers, and many subsections, not all of which are all that reasonable. It is one of these subdivisions, called the dorsolateral prefrontal cortex (dlPFC), however, that is most nearly connected to executive

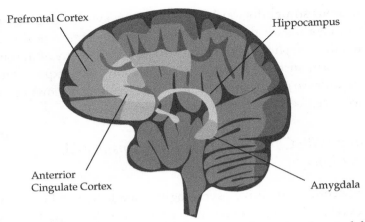

FIGURE 4 Illustration of brain regions showing the PFC and amygdala among other important areas.

Source: From https://infocenter.nimh.nih.gov

function, reason, and logic. The dlPFC is relatively shielded from the influence of more emotional parts of the brain, but readily affected by them when emotions run high. Injury to the dlPFC can result in an individual who is emotionally driven and impulsive and who has difficulty planning ahead, solving complicated problems, or understanding complex explanations.

Other parts of the PFC, however, are also critical in reasoned decision making. Frank Krueger and Jordan Grafman note that the PFC is responsible for three kinds of beliefs, all of which are fairly sophisticated:

> Neuroimaging studies of belief processing in healthy individuals and clinical studies suggest that the specific region in the most evolved part of the brain, the prefrontal cortex, may mediate three components of normal belief processing: a deliberative process of "doxastic inhibition" to reason about a belief as if it might not be true; an intuitive "feeling of rightness" about the truth of a belief; and an intuitive "feeling of wrongness" (or warning) about out-of-the-ordinary belief content.[6]

It is this notion of "doxastic inhibition" that is invoked whenever we take a scientific stance and say "Wait a minute, what if that isn't true?" We then try to reason about something we have been told by considering the opposite point of view. Hence, when we are told

"Evidence says that eating foods containing genetically modified organisms will inhibit human genes," the PFC might mediate a scientific response such as "Wait a minute, what evidence supports that statement? Let's suppose that this statement is not true. How can we know if it is or isn't factual?"

The difficulty with such rational thinking is, as Daniel Kahneman and Amos Tversky, the fathers of behavioral economics, and their followers have noted, that using the PFC and making reasoned choices is energy-consuming and tiring. They propose that it is much easier to make quick decisions than to ponder laboriously over the right path to take. When we are faced with an emergency situation this strategy is in fact the best one: slamming on the brakes when someone darts across the road in front of your car must be done automatically and without interference from the PFC. But more primitive parts of the brain are clearly inadequate to understand complicated biology and statistical inference. Hence, the natural tendency to avoid complexity and allow less sophisticated parts of the brain to make decisions obviates the opportunity to evaluate the science involved when making health decisions. Moreover, the PFC and the limbic brain are connected by tracts that run in both directions. In general, a strong PFC can inhibit the amygdala, so that reason overcomes emotion. On the other hand, powerful amygdala activation can inhibit activity in the PFC and drive the organism to a rapid and unreasoned response.

One way to examine brain activation under different conditions is by using functional magnetic resonance imaging (fMRI). Figure 5 shows a standard magnetic resonance image of the human brain. With fMRI it is possible to see which exact parts of the brain are activated by different types of stimuli. Amitai Shenhav and Joshua D. Greene studied brain activation during fMRI while the research participants made moral judgments and concluded that "the amygdala provides an affective assessment of the action in question, whereas the [ventromedial] PFC integrates that signal with a utilitarian assessment of expected outcomes to yield 'all things considered' moral judgments."[7] In general, then, the more primitive parts of the brain, represented by the amygdala and other parts of the limbic system, make fast and emotional responses that maximize immediate reward; the PFC makes decisions on the basis of reasoning that consider long-term consequences.[8]

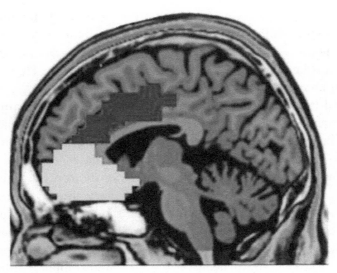

FIGURE 5 A magnetic resonance imaging (MRI) of the human brain, with two subsections of the prefrontal cortex highlighted.

Source: From J. R. van Noordt & S. J. Segalowitz, "Performance monitoring and the medial prefrontal cortex: A review of individual differences in self-regulation," *Frontiers in Human Neuroscience*, 2012, doi: 10.3389/fnhum.2012.00197.

In a fascinating series of experiments that illustrate the ways these different brain regions operate, scientists attempted to understand the neural basis of racial prejudice by showing black and white participants pictures of people of the same or opposite race. Emily Falk and Matthew D. Lieberman summarize these experiments by noting that whenever participants demonstrated a subliminal racially biased response, the amygdala was strongly activated, but when the participants were given a chance to think about their responses, the amount of amygdala activity declined and activity in the PFC increased. "Broadly speaking," they conclude, "each of these reports fit within the framework of attitude (or bias) regulation ... ; initial automatic responses in affective processing regions [e.g., the amygdala] are altered following a deliberate choice [i.e., reflected in activity in the prefrontal cortex]."[9]

Scientists are only now beginning to understand the circumstances under which one brain region dominates the other. It is clear that humans have a much greater capacity to assert reason over emotion than any other organism but that there are tremendous differences among situations and, perhaps more important, among individuals in the ability to do so. Almost all humans will run away when they smell smoke and not first try to figure out what makes smoke derive from fire. On the other hand, some people when told that nuclear power plants will inevitably leak lethal radiation into our water supply demand to know on what evidentiary basis that statement is made and others will immediately sign a petition demanding that Congress outlaw nuclear power plants.

That Good Ole Availability Heuristic

Kahneman and Tversky called the intuitive, more rapid, and less reasoned strategies that we use to make decisions *heuristics*, and show that all of us fall back on them rather than engage in more effortful reasoning when faced with complex issues. In their words, a heuristic is "a simple procedure that helps find adequate, though often imperfect, answers to difficult questions."[10]

As discussed in more detail in chapter 6 on risk perception, psychologists tell us that rather than struggling with complexity we are programmed to fall back on one of these heuristics: the *availability heuristic*. We are told by various people and organizations to worry that there is serious harm associated with gun ownership, nuclear power, genetically modified foods, antibiotics, and vaccines. But which of these should we really worry about? According to Richard H. Thaler and Cass R. Sunstein, the authors of the widely read book *Nudge*,

> In answering questions of this kind, most people used what is called the availability heuristic. They assess the likelihood of risks by asking how readily examples come to mind. If people can easily think of relevant examples, they are far more likely to be frightened and concerned than if they cannot. A risk that is familiar, like that associated with terrorism in the aftermath of 9/11, will be seen as more serious than a risk that is less familiar, like that associated with sunbathing or hotter summers. Homicides are more available than suicides, and so people tend to believe, wrongly, that more people die from homicides.[11]

Of course, orders of magnitude more people develop skin cancers, including potentially lethal types like malignant melanoma, because of sunbathing than will ever be harmed by terrorists; and of the approximately 30,000 people who are killed by guns every year in the United States, about two-thirds are suicides and one-third are murdered. Yet, we spend billions of dollars and endless hours on airport security but leave it mostly up to us to figure out which kind of sunscreen will best protect our skin from potentially fatal cancers like melanoma.

As we discuss throughout this book, heuristics such as this, that have the capacity to lead us to incorrect conclusions, most often offer important benefits and should not be viewed simply as mindless "mistakes" employed by people who lack information or are too "stupid" to understand scientific data. The availability heuristic is no different. It is imperative that we make decisions based on experience. A primitive example, of course, is that we don't touch a hot stove after once experiencing the consequences of doing so (or at least trying to do so and being screamed at by a parent "DON'T TOUCH THAT!"). If we engaged our dorsolateral prefrontal cortex every time we need to make a decision, we would be locked in place all day trying to figure things out when our own experience could give us a quick path of action. Indeed, falling back on heuristics is a normal process for several reasons. When buying groceries we can fill our basket quickly because we know pretty much what we like to eat and how much things cost. How tedious it would be if we had to engage in a project of complex reasoning every time we entered a supermarket. This kind of simple decision making based on experience and what is immediately obvious is an evolutionarily conserved and practically necessary function of our brains.

Science, however, asks us to work hard against these methods of decision making, which is why it often butts up against our psychological instincts and causes significant resistance. It is much easier for us to imagine a nuclear explosion—we have seen them in the movies countless times—than a polluted sky gradually destroying the airways of a person born with asthma. So we determine that nuclear power is more dangerous than burning coal for energy, when in fact the opposite is the case. We can all recall accidentally getting a shock from an exposed electrical wire, so we are easily convinced that shock treatment must cause brain damage, but we have no clue how electric shock can somehow stimulate a depressed person's brain to make him or her feel better, and that it is a life-saving medical procedure that should actually be employed more often.[12] In each of these cases we naturally are relying on the brain's rapid decision-making abilities that serve us so well in everyday life and generally protect us from danger. Unfortunately, however, in each case we come to the wrong conclusion.

In some instances it is quite easy to demonstrate that scientific reasoning requires tackling complexity rather than making an intuitive judgment. Steven A. Sloman uses the familiar example of the whale.[13] When we think of a whale, we first conjure an image of something that looks like a fish—it swims in the ocean and has fins. But we all know that a whale is a mammal. This is because more considered thought reminds us that whales belong to a biological classification of animals that are warm-blooded, have hair, and nurse their newborn infants. Now, although we may find the pedant at a dinner party who corrects us when we offhandedly refer to a whale as a fish to be annoying, we also agree that the correction is not controversial. A whale is a mammal. Not a big deal. On the other hand, when we are asked to imagine a nuclear power plant, the first thing that comes to mind is likely an image of the mushroom cloud over Hiroshima after the first atomic bomb was dropped in 1945. The distance from that image to an understanding of how nuclear power plants safely create huge amounts of nonpolluting energy that cannot affect the earth's ozone layer and contribute to global warming is much greater than from fish to mammals. And while almost no one harbors a meaningful fear of whales, it is natural to be frightened by anything with the word *nuclear* in it. So not only is the trip from bomb to safe power more complicated than from fish to mammal, we will naturally resist that intellectual adventure at every step because our amygdala sends off a danger signal that shuts off the prefrontal cortex and urges us, at least figuratively, to run away.

We can see clearly, then, that our fear of and retreat from complexity is mediated by powerful, evolutionarily determined aspects of human brain function that translate into psychological defaults like the availability heuristic. The question is whether it is possible to provide education that will help us overcome this fear and become confident even when scientific matters are complicated. As we will argue, based on the findings and comments of many others, traditional science education is not doing a very good job to prepare us to face up to scientific complexity. But already there is a substantial body of research pointing the way to improving this situation. We believe the basic principle to follow is to teach people, from the earliest ages possible, how science really works.

Does School Make Us Hate Science?

Americans are interested in science and technology. They visit science museums and line up to buy the latest technological gadgets. But they nevertheless think that science is too complicated for them to really understand. According to a recent Pew Foundation report, "Nearly half of Americans (46%) say that the main reason that many young people do not pursue degrees in math and science is mostly because they think these subjects are too hard."[14] Our schools' approach to teaching science appears devoted to proving this attitude correct. Americans seem prepared to throw up their hands in despair, even when they are being asked to vote on scientific issues. At the 2007 annual meeting of the American Association for the Advancement of Science (AAAS), Jon Miller presented a paper on science literacy in America. He related that in 2003 he and his colleagues at Michigan State University conducted a poll in which they ascertained the opinions of adults on a range of issues, including stem cell research. At the time, 17% were strongly in favor of such work, citing its potential for advancing cures for serious illnesses, and 17% were opposed on antiabortion grounds. Throughout the following year, stem cell research became a presidential election issue. Miller et al. repeated the poll 1 week before the election and found that now only 4% of the people backed and 4% opposed stem cell research. The rest of the people polled said the issue was just too complex.[15] We may be getting some of this inability to take a scientific "stand" from our school teachers, including high school biology teachers. When a subject like evolution is perceived as controversial in a community, Michael Berkman and Eric Plutzer of Pennsylvania State University found that science teachers are "wishy-washy" and prefer to avoid the topic altogether.[16] Of course, from the scientific point of view there is nothing remotely controversial about evolution, but we are never going to grasp that if the people charged with our scientific education are unwilling to take a strong stand on the facts.

Science education in the United States seems devoted to making people hate and fear science rather than strengthening their self-confidence in understanding complex issues. In elementary school, children are given projects to collect and label leaves that fall off trees in the fall, as if being able to differentiate an oak leaf from a maple leaf will reveal some important scientific principle. A few children enjoy getting outside and collecting leaves, but for most of them the task is pure tedium. In junior high school, biology revolves around memorizing the names of organs in pictures of insects, frogs, and dogs, as if being able to name the cloaca and the single-chambered heart will provoke an enduring love of science. By high school, the assignment might be to memorize the periodic table of the elements, all 118 of them. This includes remembering each element's atomic number, symbol, and electron configuration. How comforting for the people who someday must have an opinion on the safety of nuclear energy to know that number 118 is ununoctium. My guess is that many PhD chemists need to have the periodic table hung on the wall of their labs in order to remember all the details.

It is unfortunately the case that there is a sizeable gap between what scientists and nonscientists believe to be true about many issues, including whether it is safe to eat GMOs, vaccinate our children, or build more nuclear power plants. But it seems, as Lee Rainie recently pointed out in *Scientific American*, there is one area in which they agree: the poor state of U.S. education in science, technology, engineering, and math (the so-called STEM subjects).[17] What is important here is that demoralizing people about science from an early age biases decision making in favor of using the least energy-demanding parts of the brain. People are being conditioned to resist invoking the dlPFC and even trying to think through the scientific and health questions they must confront.

Why the Scientific Method Itself Defies Our Desire for Simplicity

Science works by something called the *scientific method*. Not infrequently we hear someone claim that they use a different scientific method than the one used by "traditional scientists." In fact, there is only one scientific method, which is actually no more controversial than saying that two plus two always equals four. The scientific method is not a matter of belief or opinion. Rather, it is a set of procedures that begins with making a hypothesis, designing and running an experiment, collecting data, analyzing the data, and reaching a conclusion about whether the results support or fail to support the original hypothesis. It is an example of *deductive reasoning*. A so-called creationist who denies the theory of evolution begins with an unfalsifiable proposition: "a higher power created the world." On the contrary, as science teacher Jacob Tanenbaum explained in an article in *Scientific American*:

> Scientists who formed the idea of human evolution did not invent the idea to go looking for fossils. Well before Charles Darwin published his treatise in 1859 and well before workers in a limestone quarry in 1856 found strange bones that would later be called Neandertal, scientists struggled to explain what they saw in the natural world and in the fossil record. The theory of evolution was the product of that analysis. That is how science works.[18]

What started as observations in nature are now the basis for understanding fundamental aspects of biology. But the process of getting there was far from simple. It is important to understand all the steps it takes to reach a scientific conclusion so that we can see clearly that "belief," emotion, and opinion should not be among them if things are done correctly.

First, Our Best Guess

There are several important steps that a scientist must take to follow the scientific method. The first one is the clear and explicit formulation of a testable hypothesis before any data gathering even begins. We stress that this hypothesis must be testable; that is, it is imperative that it can be proved wrong. It is immediately clear why the creationist's ideas cannot be considered by scientists: there is no science possible to test a hypothesis such as "God exists," because there is no experiment that can either validate or falsify such a claim. Remember, the scientific method operates by attempting to falsify hypotheses, something that seems counterintuitive at first.

For example, let us say that investigators hypothesize that an experimental drug will produce significantly more weight loss than a placebo pill. The main outcome measure is the body mass index (BMI), a measure of weight adjusted for by height. Sometimes the results of an experiment reveal something unexpected that was not part of the original hypothesis. For example, the new drug being tested for weight loss might produce more reduction in total cholesterol level than placebo. When this happens, it may prove meaningless or the harbinger of an important scientific breakthrough. But scientists cannot go back and say, "Oh, that is what I was actually looking for in the first place." Unexpected outcomes mean only one sure thing: a new experiment with a new hypothesis is in order. If the scientists want to prove the drug is also effective for cholesterol level reduction, they will have to design and conduct a new experiment with that as the main outcome measure.

The investigators' hypothesis, then, isn't "Drug is superior to placebo" but rather "There is no difference between drug and placebo." This is called the null hypothesis. They will now design and conduct an experiment to see if they can falsify or reject their null hypothesis. With the testable hypothesis in hand, the investigators must next explain exactly how they will determine whether the results of the experiment are either compatible or incompatible with it. This entails stating the study's main outcome measure. It would obviously be cheating to change the hypothesis of a study once the data start rolling in. So the investigators must state exactly what measure is the main one that will determine if the null hypothesis can be supported or rejected.

Fair and Balanced

The experimenters have decided that they will rely on weighing people and measuring how tall they are to generate the main outcome measure, BMI. But there are many more things to decide upon before starting to give people pills and asking them to get on the scale every week. The design of the experiment must be such that the hypothesis is actually being tested in a fair and balanced way. Investigators must take steps to eliminate (or at least minimize) the possibility that biases on the part of the experimenters can affect the results. Remember Yogi Berra's great line "I wouldn't have seen it if

I didn't believe it"? There are all kinds of technical details that scientists do to prevent bias from making things turn out in a preordained way, including keeping everyone involved in the experiment *blind* to which subjects are placed in which group. For example, if scientists are examining the effect that an experimental medication has on weight gain, the experimental medicine and the placebo to which it is being compared must look and taste identical and neither the scientists nor the patients can know which one they are getting. This is called a *double blind* because neither investigators nor subjects know which pill is which; this technique can be applied with certain modifications to almost every type of biological experiment.

This example also entails the important inclusion of a *control* condition. An experiment must always be constructed so that something is compared to something else. There is an experimental condition, in this case the new drug to be tested, and the control condition, here the identically appearing placebo pill. Again, the null hypothesis of this experiment is that the new drug will be no better than the placebo.

It is almost always also a requirement that subjects are *randomly assigned*, or *randomized*, to the experimental or control condition. In the weight loss study, some people will start out weighing more (that is, having a higher BMI) than others, some people will be older than others, and some people will be men. If it is the case that people who have higher BMI, are young, and are men respond preferentially to the experimental drug, then deliberately putting all such people into that group stacks the deck in favor of the experimental drug. Instead, by randomly assigning people to the two groups these differences should be evenly distributed.

A very important point with regard to proper design is adequacy of *sample size*. Because of the nature of the mathematics scientists use to analyze the data they get from their experiments, the smaller the number of subjects in a study, the more difficult it is to prove that one thing is different (or better or worse) than another even if there really is a difference. Mistakenly accepting the null hypothesis and deciding that there is no difference when in fact a difference exists is called a *Type II error*. The opposite error, declaring there is a difference when one does not really exist, is called a *Type I error*.

On the other hand, with very large sample sizes even trivial differences that will make no difference to anyone's health or life can appear to be significant from a statistical point of view. When Wakefield published his now discredited paper in *The Lancet* allegedly showing that vaccines cause autism, the first and loudest objection should have been that no such thing could possibly be proven with only 12 children as subjects. That sample size is far too small to determine if an observation is true or just chance. On the other hand, how can a large sample size give misleading results? Jack's friend and mentor, the great, late biostatistician Jacob Cohen, once wrote about an article in which it was concluded that height and IQ are positively correlated, meaning that the taller someone in the study was, the higher his or her IQ.[19] This seems a bit ridiculous. And indeed in the study, Professor Cohen noted, the sample size was so enormous that a miniscule association became statistically significant. In fact, to make a child's IQ go up 1 point, you would have to make him 1 foot taller. These details involve statistics that are not apparent to most readers but unfortunately often slip by professional reviewers and journal editors. All we can say is that 12 subjects is very small, and 10,000 is very large, and at either extreme inferences made from statistical tests of probability are prone to be misleading.

The final critical feature of a reliable experiment we wish to mention here is that the study must be both reproducible and reproduced, the latter hopefully multiple times. This means first that the experimenters have to lay out in complete detail exactly what they did, including how they picked their subjects, what tools they used to evaluate the outcomes, and how they analyzed the data. This is detailed in the Methods section in scientific papers, the part that most people skip over but is really the most important part of any paper. It must be written in such a way that other experimenters in other laboratories can replicate the exact same experiment to see if they get the same result. And the key to scientific truth is that any finding must be *replicable*: capable of being reproduced over and over again. Flukes happen in science all the time. In some cases the reasons are clear and have to do with some shortcoming in the way the initial experiment was designed or conducted. In other cases it is never clear why one researcher got one result and others another despite doing exactly the same experiment. But unless independent investigators can reproduce an experimental finding it has no value.

This is a summary of what we mean by the scientific method and the critical elements of research study design that follow from it. It is important to remember that using this method does not guarantee accurate findings. If any part of it is not done correctly the study may yield misleading or even false conclusions. But it is almost always guaranteed that if the scientific method is not followed the results of any inquiry will be useless. Scientists who use the scientific method can make mistakes; scientists who don't will almost always be wrong. And the wonderful thing about science is that mistakes are not usually replicated because no two laboratories will ever make the same exact mistake. Thus, a result that is not reproduced is automatically one to forget about entirely.

Teaching the Scientific Method

We believe that the most valuable thing students can learn in science class is how to evaluate whether or not a claim is based on evidence that has been collected by careful use of the scientific method. We also believe that an introduction to the concept of statistical inference is feasible even at the elementary school level. This does not mean, of course, trying to make fifth graders understand the details of multiple linear regression analysis. But even young children can understand concepts like chance, reproducibility, and validity. Teaching children and young adults these lessons would seem far more interesting and palatable than memorizing the names of leaves, body parts, or elements. It does not require mathematical skill, something many people (often mistakenly) claim they lack, but rather logical reasoning competence. As such, when taught properly this view of science is accessible and indeed fascinating, something that students will enjoy tackling. A recent study showed that exposing young children—in this case disadvantaged children—to high-quality, intensive interventions aimed at countering the effects of early life adverse experiences led to better health when they were adults, including a reduction in health risks like obesity.[20] The study, published in *Science*, was a carefully conducted, prospectively designed, randomized trial that meets all of the criteria we have outlined for following the scientific method rigorously. It showed that an intervention conducted from the time children are born through age 5 had a lifelong effect that included improving health behaviors. It begs the question whether interventions attempting to improve science literacy, begun at an early age, might not be capable of producing long-lived effects in a more scientifically savvy group of adults.[21] But the key element will be to emphasize process over content: how science is conducted, how scientists reach conclusions, and why some things are just chance and others are reproducible facts of nature.

How much more interesting would science class be in the fifth grade if, instead of informing the children that today in class they would be classifying a bunch of rocks into various categories of igneous, sedimentary, and metamorphic, the teacher began by asking, "Does anyone have any idea how we decide if something is true?" Other opening questions could include "What happens in a laboratory?" and "How do we know if a medicine we are given is really going to make us better?" As Sheril Kirshenbaum recently put it on CNN,

> It doesn't matter whether every American can correctly answer a pop quiz about science topics he or she had to memorize in grade school. Isn't that what turns a lot of us off to science to begin with? What's important is that we work to foster a more engaged American public that will not only support but also prioritize the research and development necessary to meet the 21st century's greatest challenges, from drought to disease pandemics.[22]

The way to defeat the fear of complexity, then, is to give people from the earliest possible ages the tools they will need to understand the scientific method.

Don't Lecture Me

Using this approach, how might a nonscientist evaluate a politically and emotionally charged issue like whether nuclear power is safe, HIV causes AIDS, ECT causes brain damage, or vaccines cause autism? How do we deal with the fact that each of these issues involves highly complex science that most people are unprepared to tackle?

One thing that should not be done is to rely solely on lectures. This includes simple lectures, complicated lectures, reassuring lectures, and frightening lectures. Instead of forcing information on people, it is better to first find out what their state of understanding is, what their goals are, and what they have been told so far. In other words, ask them questions. Studies have shown that people are far more likely to use the reasoning parts of their brains—the PFC—when they are engaged and involved in a discussion than when they are passively listening to someone else. The task here is to engage the PFC of the person we are trying to convince rather than shooting facts into the black box of an uninvolved brain. It is easy to see how a passive and disengaged person might readily default to the brain's more primitive systems, the ones that require much less effort and make emotional and impulsive judgments. It is actually possible to increase the activity of the dorsolateral PFC by training an individual in what are known as executive tasks, the ability to plan and carry out complex operations using logic and reason.[23] Doing so appears to also reduce the reactivity of the amygdala to emotional stimuli. While we are not advocating a model of human sensibility that is all reason and no emotion, there is little question that more effortful thinking about complex issues and less responding to emotionally laden sloganeering is needed if we are to be equipped with the ability to make evidence-based health decisions. Teaching the method in an ongoing way at a young age will make the whole process of interpreting scientific data for the general public much less complex and confusing and should help adults make health decisions with less mental energy and lower reliance on heuristics.

Motivating the Brain to Accept Change

Neuroscientists also tell us that changing one's viewpoint on any issue is difficult, in part because staying put with a point of view activates the pleasure centers of the brain whereas making a change excites areas of the brain associated with anxiety and even disgust. Yu and colleagues at Cambridge and University College London had subjects participate in a gambling task while their brain regional activity was measured using fMRI.[24] The game involves giving participants the chance to stick with a default position or make a change to a new position. They found that staying put activated an area of the brain called the ventral striatum whereas changing activated the insula. The ventral striatum, which includes the brain structure called the nucleus accumbens (NAc) mentioned earlier, is central to the brain's pleasure response. It is one of the parts of the brain that is routinely stimulated by drugs like alcohol and heroin and lights up in animals and people whenever they are happy. Direct stimulation of the ventral striatum with electrodes can make animals demonstrate pleasure-related responses. By contrast, the insula is activated when someone is anxious or frightened or shown disgusting pictures. In their experiment, Yu and colleagues also found that when a person loses a bet after switching, he feels worse than when he loses after staying put. So changing an opinion is associated with fear, which is precisely what we need to overcome if we are going to change people's minds from familiar, easy default positions to more complex scientific ones.

Furthermore, activity in these same brain regions mediates how a person's mood affects his or her willingness and ability to make a change. In an ultimatum game experiment, a type of economics experiment that is used to reveal how people make choices, K. M. Harlé and colleagues of the Department of Psychology at the University of Arizona observed that sad participants rejected more unfair monetary offers than participants in a neutral mood and that these sad people had increased activity in the insula and decreased activity in the ventral striatum.[25] Of course, rejecting an unfair offer is a positive outcome, so one could say that in this case feeling sad was protective. But the point of this important experiment is that unhappy people are resistant to change and this is reflected in activation of specific brain regions. Everything seems distasteful to them (anterior insula) and little evokes pleasure (ventral striatum). Anxious individuals are similarly unable to keep up with new evidence as it comes in and therefore resist updating their ideas about what is true.[26] The message here is that our countervailing messages must be stimulating and upbeat, designed to stimulate the ventral striatum rather than the insula. It is also probably best if they avoid evoking anxiety and fear. Indeed, experiments judging the effectiveness of various pro-science communications might be conducted during functional imaging. Those that most activated the striatum and least activated the anterior insula should be the ones selected for further testing as being more likely to be effective.

A model for guiding people to sort out scientific fact from fiction is a technique used by mental health professionals called motivational interviewing (MI), mentioned in passing in the previous chapter, which has been found to be particularly helpful in getting people to adopt healthy behaviors like stopping excessive alcohol intake or adhering to medication regimens for diabetes. Instead of ordering the patient to stop drinking or take the medicine, the clinician attempts to motivate the patient to do these things by collaboratively assessing what it is that the patient hopes to achieve. An alcoholic patient may begin by insisting she doesn't want to stop drinking, but agree that she does want to stop getting arrested for DWIs. The diabetic patient may initially say the medications are a nuisance and he doesn't feel sick anyway, but he may also express a wish to avoid having a heart attack in the next few years. By first establishing what goals the patient has, the interviewer can then proceed to work with him or her on how to achieve them.

In a similar manner, one approach to dealing with the complexity problem may be to begin by establishing what goals and values individuals have. In some instances, like when a clinician discusses vaccines, ECT, or antibiotic use with a patient, this can be done on an individual, face-to-face basis. In others, such as decisions about nuclear power or GMOs, it will be necessary to design public health approaches that can engage larger populations. Here are some goals with which most people on either side of some of the issues we are dealing with in this book will likely agree:

1. *Vaccines:* I want to make sure my children are as protected as possible from preventable infectious diseases, and I want other children in my community to have the same protection.

2. *Antibiotics:* I want only medication that is known to be effective for an illness that I or a member of my family might have, and I don't want medication that poses a greater risk to health than a benefit.

3. *ECT:* If someone is severely depressed to the point that her life is in danger because she is not eating or might resort to suicide, I think she should have treatment that is most likely to reduce the depression without causing severe, irreversible adverse effects.

4. *GMOs:* A technology with which I am not familiar, even if it has been in use for decades, is something about which I will always be cautious and even skeptical. I need to be convinced in

terms I understand that it is safe. I do agree that helping to alleviate hunger and starvation around the world is a worthwhile goal, but not at the cost of harming my family.

5. *Nuclear power:* We need cheaper, cleaner sources of energy that won't pollute the air and add to the problem of global warming.

6. *HIV as the cause of AIDS:* AIDS is a terrible disease, and it is important to know what causes it so that effective treatments can be developed. The issue is how scientists establish what causes an illness and whether in the case of AIDS they have actually done so.

7. *Gun ownership:* I want to protect my home and my family from anyone or anything that might try to harm us, including intruders in my home. But I don't allow things in my home that could harm me or my family.

8. *Pasteurization:* It is important to me that my family consumes foods that have high nutritional content and low risk for causing infectious or other medical problems.

Starting with these premises, the process develops along Socratic lines in which the interviewer assesses at each step what the interviewee knows and has heard about the topic and what he or she wants to know. Let us take the first case, vaccines, as an example. First let us describe a well-meant example of what probably is not going to work. Sam Wang is a neuroscientist at Princeton University who has worked in the area of finding causes for autism. His March 29, 2014, op-ed piece in *The New York Times* titled "How to Think About the Risk of Autism" is clearly written, informative, and convincing. He urges us to think in terms of a statistical measure called "risk ratio," which he says is "a concept we are familiar with." The higher the risk ratio, the higher the risk. He points out that the risk ratio for vaccines and autism is less than 1.0, meaning there is absolutely no risk of vaccines causing autism. On the other hand, elective cesarean section has a risk ratio for autism of 1.9, meaning that people who have been born via cesarean section have nearly twice the rate of developing autism than people born by vaginal delivery. He cites risk ratios for several other factors, some larger than others, and also points out the following:

The human genome is dotted with hundreds of autism risk genes. Individually, each gene is usually harmless, and is in fact essential for normal function. This suggests that autism is caused by combinations of genes acting together. Think of genes as being like playing cards, and think of autism outcomes as depending on the entire hand. New mutations can also arise throughout life, which might account for the slightly greater risk associated with older fatherhood.

The problem here is that Wang's article is loaded with information about genetic and environmental causes of autism. We are told about hundreds of risk genes, a concept that is not immediately intuitive to the nonspecialist. Most people have heard of genes that cause diseases, like Huntington's disease, but the concept of multiple risk genes that are somehow normal until they combine in a certain way, while biologically plausible, is difficult to grasp. On top of that, a bevy of other risk ratios for causes of autism are given, including the cesarean section risk mentioned earlier, plus maternal stress both before and after pregnancy, air pollution, lack of social stimulation, and damage to the cerebellum at birth. Wang concludes, "When reading or watching the news, remember that scare stories are not always what they seem. In this respect, looking at the hard data can help parents keep a cool head."[27]

But in fact, Wang's article is scary. Instead of clinging to the false idea that vaccines cause autism, Wang is now telling parents that hundreds of their genes may be causing the problem and that the reason they have a child with autism may be that the mother was anxious during pregnancy and had an elective cesarean section. How stress and cesarean sections might cause autism is probably not a lot more obvious to parents of children with autism than the multiple genes theory. Wang means to write for a general audience, and indeed *New York Times's* readers probably have above average intelligence. But his explanations sound complicated, and elucidating them would require a great deal of explanation. The way in which genes can interact to cause a disease is, in fact, a very complicated process. So is the mechanism by which stress can alter the development of a fetal brain. Once again, a passive reader may readily default to the emotionally much easier position that a poisonous substance in vaccines, thimerosal, causes autism. It is easier to grasp the notion that something toxic added to our bodies causes a serious problem than that multiple genes we already have combine in mystical ways to do us harm.

We do not mean here to criticize Wang's article, which is an honest attempt at explaining why the autism/vaccine notion is unfounded. He is trying very hard to explain to the nonscientist why this is the case, and we applaud him and every scientist who makes an honest effort to do so. Wang never condescends to his reader, nor does he imply we are not smart enough to understand what he is saying. Our point is, however, that the audience's state of mind must always first be understood. If that state is one of anxious concern and fear, as is the case for many parents trying to decide if it is okay to vaccinate their children, substituting misinformation with new facts is not guaranteed to change minds. The groundwork first needs to be laid to create a receptive, calm audience that is open to considering new ideas. Adapting the techniques of MI is an approach we believe can accomplish this and should be studied in that context.

Starting at the Right Place

The key, then, is to use motivational interviewing techniques to change the passive listener of scientific information into an active participant in a scientific discussion. In the aforementioned studies reviewed by Falk and Lieberman about brain activation during the expression of racial prejudice it was noted that amygdala activation associated with bias "disappeared when participants were required to verbally label the images as belonging to a given race, and the amount of increased activity in right [ventrolateral prefrontal cortex] correlated with a decrease in amygdala activity."[28] Simply put, talking out loud about our biases engages our executive brain and reduces fear. This is the first step in a more reasoned and less prejudiced response. The MI approach to scientific literacy begins at whatever level the interviewee (or group of people) finds him- or herself at the start of the process and can proceed to greater complexity once he or she is ready. Here is an example of how this might work:

> A nurse in a pediatrician's office is discussing vaccinating a new mother's 2-year-old child for measles, mumps, and rubella (MMR). He has established the first premise, that Ms. Jones obviously does not want her son, Douglas, to catch a dangerous disease that could be prevented and that she prides herself on being a good citizen who wants the best for all children.

The nurse, Anthony, begins the conversation by asking, "What have you heard about vaccine safety?"

"I have heard many very disturbing things," Ms. Jones replies. "I have heard many times that vaccines cause autism and other neurological problems. I also read that giving so many vaccines to children like we do now stresses the immune system of a young child and has serious consequences as they grow up."

"Let's start with the idea that vaccines cause autism. What is the basis for this claim as far as you know?"

"Ever since they started putting mercury into vaccines to preserve them, the rate of autism has gone up and up."

"Well, you are certainly right that the rate of autism in some parts of the world has increased at an alarming rate in recent years. But as you know, children had autism before they started putting mercury in vaccines, so that couldn't be the only reason."

"Right, but it does explain the increase."

"But would it change your thinking on this to know that most vaccines no longer have mercury in them but the rate of autism has continued to increase?"

"I didn't know that, but it would be hard to explain the increase if it keeps happening even when mercury is removed."

This conversation continues as Ms. Jones becomes more and more engaged. She is an active participant and with each step, Anthony is able to explain things with a bit more complexity. Eventually, he is even able to give Ms. Jones some pretty complicated explanations about the lack of biological plausibility for vaccines as a cause of autism, the danger in thinking that an association—or correlation—between two things means one caused the other,[29] and the way in which a vaccine stimulates a very small part of the human immune system in a highly specific way. Notice also that Anthony asks Ms. Jones what information she would need to make a decision when he inquires if it would change her thinking "to know that most vaccines no longer have mercury in them." An important feature here is to establish what the interviewee's level of evidence is on any topic and even to establish how she would go about gathering that information. Ask, for example, "What would it take to convince you one way or the other about vaccine safety? Let's say that one person told you about research showing a link between vaccines and autism. Would that be convincing? What credentials does that person have to have? Would you want to hear the same thing from more than one person?" It is also very important to ask the interviewee what she thinks would happen if she is wrong in her decision. "Now," Nurse Anthony might ask, "you say that you think vaccines will harm your child and you are considering taking a philosophical exemption and not having him vaccinated. Suppose, for a moment, you are wrong and vaccines don't really have anything to do with autism. What would happen then? What would be the outcome of your decision?"

There are of course problems with the scenario we have outlined. First, even in the face-to-face situation, it takes more time than healthcare professionals can often spend with each patient to play out. Second, since we assume that the pediatrician definitely does not have time for such a lengthy conversation, we assigned the task of interviewer to a nurse. But nurses are also extremely busy healthcare professionals who may not have the time for such a lengthy encounter. Third, under our often counterproductive way of funding healthcare, no reimbursement is likely available for the doctor or nurse to spend time convincing someone to vaccinate a child. Finally, this is obviously not a public health solution. It will take creativity and perhaps new insights to transfer a motivational interviewing schema into something that can be accomplished on a large population scale. But it is certainly plausible that new technologies, particularly social media, could be engineered to accomplish such a task.

We would also like to add that our lament about the lack of funding for vaccine-related counseling could be addressed. Saad Omer, an epidemiologist at Emory University, was recently quoted in a wonderful op-ed piece by Catherine Saint Louis: "Doctors should be paid separately for vaccine counseling in cases where a 'substantial proportion of time is being spent on vaccines.' "[30] Perhaps it is time to challenge the mantra "Insurance won't pay for that" every time someone comes up with a good idea for improving the public's health. After all, isn't it worth some health insurance company money to prevent needless death from diseases for which we have vaccines?

Most important, our suggested approach substitutes passive listening with active engagement and introduces complexity only as the participant becomes increasingly more engaged in the topic. It does not guarantee that the outcome will be acceptance of the scientific solution to any issue; indeed, the approach itself is testable.

Experiments can be designed to adjudicate whether a motivational approach works better than a lecture approach in convincing people to accept the outcome of the scientific method.

"Pls Visit My Website, Thanks!!!!"

We've spent a lot of time discussing academic articles and how to tell whether an article is credible or not. But more often in this day and age, we get our information from the Internet. So how can we know if a website is credible? There are no absolute rules, as this is a much freer and less developed mode of publication than that represented by peer-reviewed scientific publications. Nevertheless, we offer a few guidelines to use the next time you are searching for information on a hotly contested and confusing scientific topic.

1. *Spelling and grammar:* Obvious errors are relatively easy to spot, and most of you probably do not give much credence to websites with many errors. Yet it is still worth reiterating that if a website is very poorly written and riddled with errors, it is probably not a reliable source of information. The only exception to this is if the website is from a foreign country and/or has been translated into English.
2. *Domain:* Websites with the domains ".edu" and ".gov" are very often reliable sources of scientific information. When in doubt, look for sources with these domain names. They are your safest bet. Of course this is not to say that other domains, such as ".com," ".org," and ".net" are definitely unreliable—far from it. However, if you are really in a bind and having a hard time figuring out what's what in a scientific debate, your best bet is to look for ".edu" and ".gov" domains for reliable explanations.
3. *Sources:* Pay attention to what kinds of sources the articles or information on the website cite. Do they make a lot of claims without citing any sources at all? Unless it's a purely and explicitly opinion-based website, this is usually a bad sign. If they do cite sources, try to do a little investigation. What kinds of sources are they? Do they simply link to very similar websites with no sources listed? Or do they take you to a wide array of peer-reviewed, scientific journal articles? Also pay attention to

how dated the cited material is. Science moves very quickly, and if a website is consistently citing information from many, many years ago, that is a good sign that it is not a reliable source.

4. *Design:* This is of course very subjective, but in general, reliable websites have a certain professional look and feel to them. They are usually relatively well designed (although government agencies with tight budgets may not be too fancy). The website should at the very least look neat and nicely organized. Clutter, excessive use of exclamation marks, large and multi-colored fonts, and graphic photos are all good indications of an unreliable website.

5. *Author information:* When materials on the website include an author's name, take a moment to research him or her. What is that person's web presence? Does a quick Google search bring up 37 petitions signed by this person against GMOs and a picture of him or her at an anti-GMO rally? Or does it yield a professional website with evidence of expertise in the area in question? This is a very important and quick way to measure whether the website is trying to bias you in a certain direction and, more important, whether its information is accurate and authoritative.

Now let's do a little exercise. First look at figure 6, close the book, and write down as many red flags as you can.

How did you do? We counted at least five red flags: graphic photos (especially the one of the baby being stuck by many needles), multiple colors and fonts with random bolding and spacing, clutter, inappropriate exclamatory statements ("Smallpox Alert!"), and, although you cannot tell from the photo, distracting graphics, since many of the elements of the homepage are actually moving, flashing graphics. Now compare this homepage to the homepage in figure 7.

Figure 7 is the CDC's homepage on vaccination and immunizations. Now, this might not be the most beautiful website you've ever seen, but it is clean, organized, and consistent in its use of fonts, bolding, and color. It has no flashing graphics or distracting exclamation points. This is a website we can trust. While this is no fool-proof method, the guidelines provided earlier should enable you to evaluate the claims of any given website. Even if the website cites

Vaccination Liberation - Home

* "Free Your Mind....From The Vaccine Paradigm"

#Great Vaccination Quotes: | List of Random Quotes

And my experience is that the ordinary intelligent anti-vaccinator can dumbfound nine-tenths of the medical men on the subject.
W. R.HADWEN, M.D., J.P. 1902

Scary diseases do not justify scary vaccines. - Dewy Duffel

Legal/Help:	Science:	Misc:	Searches:
*Exemption Page	Introduction	Membership	KeyWord Index
*Resource Contacts/Help	Basic Facts | Q and A	Books Videos Tapes	Search Our Site
Avoid Vaccinations	Package Inserts	*Testimonies	Contact Us
Activism	Ingredients of Vaccines	Español—VacLib	
LegalNews	Artificially Sweetened Times	News	Finding Pediatricians
	Smallpox Alert!	Planned Events	

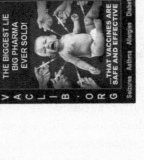

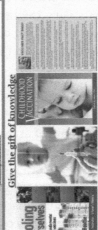

Give the gift of knowledge

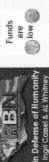

Funds are low

FIGURE 6 Vaccination Liberation Group homepage (http://www.vaclib.org).

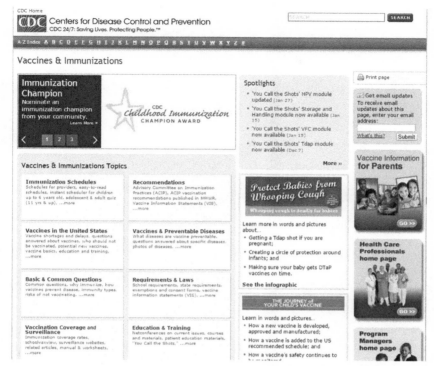

FIGURE 7 CDC Vaccine & Immunizations homepage (http://www.cdc.gov/vaccines/).

100 scientific articles, paying attention to small details like design and imagery can help you distinguish what's true from what might simply be misinformed, if not bogus.

It is clearly urgent that we bridge the gap between what the scientific community has learned and what nonscientists know, or think they know, about scientific advances. This gulf will at times seem vast, and there is no possible appeal to have the waters split and knowledge diffuse broadly through the population. The process will not succeed if smart people think the solution is to hector, deride, or condescend to us. We need an experimental approach to the transfer of scientific knowledge, one that follows all of the principles of the scientific method involved in acquiring this knowledge in the first place.

Risk Perception and Probability

EACH DAY, WHEN YOU TAKE YOUR MORNING SHOWER, YOU face a 1 in 1,000 chance of serious injury or even death from a fall. You might at first think that each time you get into the shower your chance of a fall and serious injury is 1 in 1,000 and therefore there is very little to worry about. That is probably because you remember that someone once taught you the famous coin-flip rule of elementary statistics: because each toss is an independent event, you have a 50% chance of heads each time you flip. But in this case you would be wrong. The actual chance of falling in the shower is additive. This is known in statistics as the "law of large numbers." If you do something enough times, even a rare event will occur. Hence, if you take 1,000 showers you are almost assured of a serious injury—about once every 3 years for a person who takes a shower every day. Of course, serious falls are less common than that because of a variety of intervening factors. Nevertheless, according to the CDC, mishaps near the bathtub, shower, toilet, and sink caused an estimated 234,094 nonfatal injuries in the United States in 2008 among people at least 15 years old.[1]

In 2009, there were 10.8 million traffic accidents and 35,900 deaths due to road fatalities in the United States.[2] The CDC estimates a 1-in-100 lifetime chance of dying in a traffic accident and a 1-in-5 lifetime chance of dying from heart disease. But none of these realities affect our behaviors very much. We don't take very many (if any) precautions when we shower. We text, eat, talk on the phone, and zone out while driving, paying little attention to the very real risk we pose to ourselves (and others) each time we get in the car. And we keep eating at McDonald's and smoking cigarettes, completely disregarding the fact that these behaviors could eventually affect our health in extreme and fatal ways.

On the other hand, there is *zero* proven risk of death as a result of the diphtheria-tetanus-pertussis (DTP) vaccine. But the death rate from diphtheria is 1 in 20 and the death rate from tetanus is a whopping 2 in 10.[3] Yet we are seeing an unprecedented decrease in numbers of parents opting to vaccinate their children across the developed world. One in four U.S. parents still believes that vaccines cause autism, although this theory has been thoroughly debunked.[4] Twenty-one U.S. states now allow "philosophical exemptions" for those who object to vaccination on the basis of personal, moral, or other beliefs. In recent years, rates of philosophical exemptions have increased, rates of vaccination of young children have decreased, and resulting infectious disease outbreaks among children have been observed in places such as California and Washington. In California, the rate of parents seeking philosophical exemptions rose from 0.5% in 1996 to 1.5% in 2007. Between 2008 and 2010 in California, the number of kindergarteners attending schools in which 20 or more children were intentionally unvaccinated nearly doubled: from 1,937 in 2008 to 3,675 in 2010.[5] These facts prompted California to eliminate the philosophical objections option recently, although it is unclear whether this welcome change in the law is accompanied by a change in the views of those California parents who took advantage of the option while it was still available. Vaccination rates have also decreased all over Europe,[6] resulting in measles and rubella outbreaks in France, Spain, Italy, Germany, Switzerland, Romania, Belgium, Denmark, and Turkey. In 2013, there was a devastating outbreak of 1,000 cases of measles in Swansea, Wales, that has been traced to parental fears about vaccination that are directly related to Andrew Wakefield's 1998 paper (erroneously claiming) that vaccines cause autism.[7]

Don't Let the Data Get in Your Way?

A similar dynamic can be seen in public notions of the risks associated with guns. The actual lifetime odds of dying as a result of assault with a firearm are estimated to be about 1 in 325. Fearing an armed invasion is a leading reason that people make the decision to keep a gun in the house. Remember that posting by the pro-gun organization Heartland depicting an actress claiming to have a gun for protection that we discussed in chapter 3? A famous actress confidently tells us that she has a gun and will defend her children from armed invaders. Yet that a gun in the home is more likely to kill someone who lives there than an intruder is an indisputable fact.[8] In 2003 Douglas Wiebe, then at UCLA and now at the University of Pennsylvania, reported the results of two large studies clearly showing that having a gun at home increases the risk of being murdered or killing oneself.[9] Several years later, Wiebe's research group found that having a gun makes a person more than 4 times more likely to be shot during an assault compared to people without guns.[10] Thus, even trying to defend oneself with a gun is more likely to get the gun owner killed than it is to stop an assailant. Harvard's David Hemenway points out that "in three national self-defense gun surveys sponsored by the Harvard Injury Control Research Center, no one reported an incident in which a gun was used to protect a child under fourteen."[11] Kellerman and Mercy analyzed homicides of women between 1976 and 1987 and found that half were killed by people they knew or by their husbands whereas only 13% were killed by strangers.[12] Although it may be true that there are instances in which a person with a gun successfully uses it to protect himself from an assailant, this is clearly the exception. It may be that there are some instances in which not wearing a seat belt saved a life that would have been lost had the driver been wearing one, but no one denies the clear evidence that wearing a seat belt makes us safer. According to the American Academy of Pediatrics, "The absence of guns from homes and communities is the most effective measure to prevent suicide, homicide, and unintentional injuries to children and adolescents."[13] Overall, having a gun makes a person less safe. Despite all of the incontrovertible facts just cited, gathered by careful, objective scientific research, about 37% of Americans have guns at home for self-protection.[14]

So why do we ignore the considerable risks associated with everyday activities like showering and driving, while we fret over the very small to nonexistent likelihood of our children reacting adversely to a vaccination or of an intruder bursting into our homes and shooting us dead? The answer, we believe, lies in the psychology of risk perception. Both vaccines and guns involve two kinds of misguided risk assessment: denial of real risks and simultaneous acceptance of unrealistic, false, or small risks. In the case of vaccines, parents who refuse to vaccinate their children are both denying the real risk of the horrendous infectious diseases that were once responsible for overwhelming numbers of childhood deaths and believing as substantial a nearly zero risk of neurological damage or death from vaccines. In the case of guns, gun owners are denying the accumulated risk of suicide or homicide by a family member that accompanies having a gun in the home and exaggerating a very small risk of being killed in a firearm assault. From these examples we suggest that when it comes to health, people are intolerant of risks of harm that feel uncontrollable while they are perfectly content to accept risks that they perceive are within their control, even if these perceptions are incorrect. For example, everyone who drives *believes* he or she is a safe driver and totally in control of what happens on the road. In fact, 90% of drivers think they are better than average, which is, of course, statistically nearly impossible.[15] In much the same way, many people who own guns seem positive that no one in *their* family will ever become suicidal or suddenly so enraged that he or she might turn the gun on him- or herself or someone else. Those things, they may think, occur only in other families. These particular dangerous health misperceptions fall under the psychological category we call *uncontrollable risk*. We don't make the vaccines ourselves, someone else does, and because that manufacturer is out of our direct control, we think something could be wrong with them. In this chapter, we explore the question of why many statistically improbable risks seem much more relevant to us than statistically probable ones. We begin with an overview of classic risk perception theory, discuss some of the reasons we misperceive probabilities, look at some of the heuristics and biases that affect risk perception, and conclude as always with suggestions for living by the evidence.

We Can't Always Tell What's Risky

There are a few central reasons, relevant to the way we think, process information, and often make cognitive mistakes, that explain why we so frequently misjudge risk. The first is that people tend to be poor at interpreting probabilities. Even people who are well trained in statistics often falter when interpreting risk probabilities, especially when emotions are involved, as in the case of deciding whether to vaccinate your children. In addition, the way probabilities are framed in many ways determines people's perceptions of the relevance of the risk and its extent. Risk perception is particularly prone to change based on the *type* of risk (short-term versus long-term, individual-level versus population-level, etc.), so our estimates are not always based purely on the quantitative aspects associated with the real probability of incurring the risk. Finally, risk perception is a fundamentally social phenomenon and is extremely sensitive to group dynamics and social cues. Risk perception in groups is therefore often different from risk perception in individuals. All of these features of risk and the way we process it can lead us down the wrong path, misunderstanding the consequences of particular actions and sometimes causing us to make the wrong decisions. As Nobel laureate Daniel Kahneman put it, "When called upon to judge probability, people actually judge something else and believe they have judged probability."[16]

Early research on risk perception assumed that people assess risk in a "rational" manner, weighing information before making a decision, the way scientists do (or at least are supposed to do). This approach assumes that providing people with more information will alter their perceptions of risk. Subsequent research has demonstrated that providing more information alone will not assuage people's irrational fears and sometimes outlandish ideas about what is truly risky. The psychological approach to risk perception theory, championed by psychologist Paul Slovic, examines the particular heuristics (i.e. simple methods that people use to solve difficult problems) and biases people invent to interpret the amount of risk in their environment.

In *Science* in 1987, Slovic summarized various social and cultural factors that lead to inconsistent evaluations of risk by the general public.[17] Slovic emphasizes the essential way in which experts' and laypeople's views of risk differ. Experts judge risk in terms of quantitative assessments of morbidity and mortality. Yet most people's perception of risk is far more complex, involving numerous psychological and cognitive processes. Slovic's review demonstrates the complexity of our assessment of risk. As we alluded to earlier, no matter how many numbers we throw at people, we still think that only what we aren't in control of can hurt us. This is a little like a child who thinks once he is in bed and closes his eyes the monsters can't get him any longer. You cannot convince the child that monsters don't exist or that closing his eyes is not a defense against an attack by telling him what the prevalence of monsters or monster attacks are in each state in the United States. But that is probably the approach a scientist would take. A better approach, and one we will come back to in a moment, is that of the loving parent who has gained the child's trust and is able to reassure him that monsters don't come into the house.

Perhaps more important than quantifying our responses to various risks is to identify the qualitative characteristics that lead us to specific valuations of risk. Slovic masterfully summarizes the key qualitative characteristics that result in judgments that a certain activity is risky or not. Besides being intolerant of risks that we perceive as uncontrollable, we cannot tolerate risks that might have catastrophic potential, have fatal consequences, or involve one group taking a risk and a separate group reaping the benefits. Slovic notes that nuclear weapons and nuclear power score high on all of these characteristics. That is, (1) we don't control what happens inside of a nuclear power plant; (2) if there actually is a nuclear accident it could be fatal; and (3) we get electricity anyway, so how is it worth the risk to try to get it from nuclear power plants? An epidemiologist might counter that (a) catastrophic nuclear accidents are rare (we hear about freak accidents like Chernobyl and Fukushima only once every few decades), (b) there are safeguards built into modern plants, and (c) even if there is an accident, the consequences are less likely to result in substantial numbers of human casualties (to be sure, nuclear power still poses a variety of safety risks, which is a very good reason to speed up research into how to make them safer, not to condemn them outright). The climatologist might further point out that the way we currently make electricity is destroying the environment and will ultimately result in all kinds of catastrophes like melting solar ice caps, polar bears stranded on floating shards of ice, and floods that destroy property and take lives. In fact, global warming is already producing an increase in devastating storms like Superstorm Sandy and Typhoon Haiyan, leading to a much greater loss of life than anything imaginable from nuclear power. And although this may at first seem counterintuitive, from a health perspective nuclear power is clearly a safer source of energy than the coal, oil, and gas we now use to produce most of our electricity.[18]

But to a nonscientist, statistics on nuclear accidents and warnings about global warming seem remote and impersonal. A nuclear power plant exploding and killing everyone within 1,000 miles is somehow more graspable and therefore more to be feared.

Also unbearable are risks that are unknown, new, and delayed in their manifestation of harm. These factors tend to be characteristic of chemical technologies. The higher a hazard scores on these factors, the higher its perceived risk and the more people want to see the risk reduced.

Slovic's analysis goes a long way in explaining why we persist in maintaining extreme fears of nuclear energy while being relatively unafraid of driving automobiles, even though the latter has caused many more deaths than the former. The risk seems familiar and knowable. There is also a low level of media coverage of automobile accidents, and this coverage never depicts future or unknown events resulting from an accident. There is no radioactive "fallout" from a car crash. On the other hand, nuclear energy represents an unknown risk, one that cannot be readily analyzed due to a relative lack of information. Nuclear accidents evoke widespread media coverage and warnings about possible future catastrophes. A mysterious thing called "radiation" can cause damage many years after the actual accident. While it is easy to understand what happens when one car crashes into another and heads are pushed through windshields, most people don't really know what radiation is. What is that business about the decay of atomic nuclei releasing subatomic particles that can cause cancer? In this case, a lower risk phenomenon (nuclear energy) actually induces much more fear than a higher risk activity (driving an automobile). It is a ubiquitous human characteristic to overestimate small probabilities (the reason people continue to buy lottery tickets even though there is really no chance of winning) and underestimate large possibilities (enabling us to blithely continue to consume more calories than we can burn off). Perhaps even more striking are recent findings that Macaque monkeys are prone to exactly the same risk perception distortions as we humans are.[19] The authors of that study suggest that this finding demonstrates an evolutionarily conserved bias toward distorting probabilities that stretches back millions of years to our nonhuman primate ancestors.

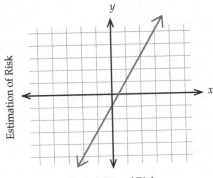

FIGURE 8 Linear probability model.

From a technical point of view, psychologists, behavioral economists, and neuroscientists call the tendency of people to overestimate small probabilities and underestimate large ones *nonlinear estimation of probability*. If we make a plot diagram (see figure 8) in which estimation of risk is on the vertical (*y*) axis and actual probability is on the horizontal (*x*) axis, a completely rational result (called *utilitarian* by economists) would be a straight diagonal line with a slope of 1. That is, the greater the actual chance of something bad happening, the greater our perception of the risk. Because this ideal results in a straight line on our plot diagram, it is called a linear response. In fact, numerous experiments have shown that the real-life plot diagram is nonlinear: small probabilities on the left side of the horizontal axis have higher than expected risk perception, and high probabilities on the right side of the horizontal axis have unexpectedly lower risk perceptions (see figure 9).

Our brains are actually hardwired for these kinds of skewed risk perceptions. As we have noted, the part of the brain in animals and humans that is activated in response to an anticipated reward is called the ventral striatum. In a fascinating experiment, Ming Hsu and colleagues performed brain imaging using functional magnetic resonance imaging (fMRI) to examine activation of the striatum while subjects performed a gambling task.[20] They found that when participants had different probabilities of getting a reward from gambling, the strength of ventral striatum activation followed the exact same nonlinear pattern as is predicted by the psychological experiments

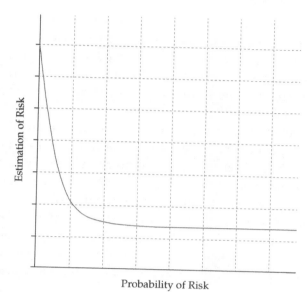

FIGURE 9 Nonlinear estimation of risk.

described earlier. In other words, our brains force this nonlinear risk assessment habit on us.

Many risk theorists, coming from an academic tradition based in psychology, have noted that calculations of risk probabilities rely heavily on emotions and affective judgments. This is one of the ways in which individuals making risk assessments on a daily basis differ so radically from expert risk assessors, who rely exclusively on numbers and probabilities, and why their judgments of the risk involved in the same activity or phenomenon can be so divergent. For example, Slovic and others examined risk attitudes of residents of an area with frequent disastrous floods. Their research uncovered several distinct "systematic mechanisms" for dealing with the uncertainty that accompanies living in an area of pervasive high risk. Some people viewed floods as repetitive or cyclical events and thus afforded them a kind of regularity that they did not actually display. Another common strategy was to invoke what the researchers termed "the law of averages," in which people tended to believe that the occurrence of a severe flood in one year meant that it was unlikely for a severe flood to occur in the following year. In fact, there is no natural reason that severe flooding needs to follow such a pattern. Other residents simply engaged in a form of flat-out denial. Some believed they were protected by newfangled "protective devices" that actually had no ability to protect them from severe flooding. Others seemed to have formed the belief that past floods were due to a "freak combination of circumstances" that were exceedingly unlikely to recur together in the future.[21]

Slovic and colleagues found that "ease of imagination" played a large role in public perceptions of risk. For example, the researchers found a heightened sense of public concern over the risks of injury and death from attack by a grizzly bear in North American national parks. In fact, the rate of injury from a grizzly bear attack is only 1 per 2 million visitors, with the death rate even smaller and thus, statistically speaking, negligible. Yet the ability to imagine the adverse event, due to the availability of photos from newspaper reporting, seems to have amplified the *perception* of risk for many people.[22]

Familiarity Breeds Errors

In terms of what *types* of risks are tolerated by most people, it seems that familiarity and the perceived tradeoff of risks and benefits are paramount. We tend to tolerate risks that are familiar, frequently encountered, or part of a well-understood system. This, risk theorists contend, goes a long way in explaining why we do not regard trains as high risk, even shortly after news of a highly publicized wreck, but a small accident in a nuclear reactor will cause significant social disturbance and heightened fear and avoidance of nuclear technologies. Risk theorists propose that we make this distinction in our minds based on the familiarity of the system in which the accident occurred. In other words, our brains are taking advantage of a common heuristic, or shortcut: familiar is good and safe; unfamiliar is bad and dangerous. This crude dichotomy, with which we all engage and probably rely on more heavily than we realize, is not entirely illogical and likely allows us to make good decisions when we are faced with potential threats and little time to decide how to deal with them. This heuristic is useful, for example, in helping us to realize that we can most likely safely approach a familiar dog in our neighborhood but that we might want to keep our distance from an unfamiliar stray dog that may be aggressive or diseased.

In a way, this reliance on the familiar to make risk judgments is not irrational at all. As Kasperson notes, direct experience with something, such as driving a car, can provide us with feedback on the "nature, extent, and manageability of the hazard, affording better perspective and enhanced capability for avoiding risks."[23] The problem is that sometimes we rely too heavily on our heuristics and misinterpret information about the true nature of the risk we are confronting. Sometimes a reliance on familiarity is a good way to judge threats when we must make a decision in a split second (e.g., Should I run away from an unfamiliar creature charging toward me?). The trouble is that we sometimes use these heuristics in contexts in which they are not entirely appropriate. A simple heuristic of familiarity or unfamiliarity may work perfectly well when deciding whether to approach or stay away from a strange dog on our front lawn, but it does not when the issue is the safety of nuclear power, an extremely complex issue that requires hours of research and discussions with experts to even begin to understand. Paradoxically, the more information we are bombarded with, the more we rely on these heuristics. It therefore makes sense that a large volume of information flow is often associated with the amplification of risk.[24] The next few sections of this chapter will be devoted to examining those situations in which we inappropriately use heuristics and mental biases in risk assessments and end up misjudging the true nature and salience of the threat.

Compared to What?

The issue of the safety of nuclear power or vaccines also raises something we refer to as the "Compared to what?" issue. If all you know is that there were 50 excess cancer deaths from the Chernobyl nuclear power reactor disaster in the 20 years after the explosion, you would be justified in saying that is too many—in modern society we believe that we should try to prevent every premature death possible and that every life has enormous intrinsic value. Yet when we point out that this death rate is a fraction of the deaths caused by other forms of energy in widespread use, like electricity derived from burning fossils fuels, the situation completely changes and nuclear power actually appears to be a legitimate alternative that we must consider.[25] Instead of calling for a ban on nuclear power plants, we should follow the lead of the Union of Concerned Scientists, which calls for funding to put in place better safety and security measures at nuclear energy facilities, steps to bring the price down for building new plants, and more research into tricky areas like safe nuclear waste disposal.[26] The enormity of the gun problem in the United States is made much more palpable when it is compared to something else: the number of deaths in the United States annually from guns is almost equal to the number from automobile accidents (more than 30,000). Our minds don't automatically ask the question "Compared to what?" when someone tells us the probability of something bad happening. Rather, we are programmed to respond to the emotional content of the presentation. Someone who somberly declares that "50 people died needlessly because of Chernobyl" gets our attention, especially if that is accompanied by pictures of corpses, atomic mushroom clouds, and the corporate headquarters of a nuclear power company.

We Probably Don't Understand Probability

Part of the reason it is often so difficult to effectively assess risk is that understanding risk depends heavily on understanding probabilities, and, for a number of psychological reasons, most people, including expert statisticians and scientists, are not very good at understanding probabilities on an intuitive level. In our everyday thinking, our minds are much more comfortable with individual narratives than with broad, population-based figures. We readily consume and make sense of anecdotes and experiences, but we struggle with likelihoods and other percentages. This is in part because it is very difficult for us to imagine events that have never happened, to think concretely about things that are not immediately tangible, and to sit comfortably with uncertainty.

Our brains have an enormous incentive to do away with uncertainty, which is why we all form such myriad and often sophisticated heuristics and biases to help us form judgments, develop opinions, and project into the future. Probabilities require us to think about two universes: one in which one event occurs (e.g., my child gets vaccinated and is healthy) and one in which another, counterfactual, event occurs (e.g., my child gets vaccinated and has an adverse reaction). Neither one of these universes exists in the present, the moment at which the child actually gets the shot or swallows the vaccine; furthermore, once the first universe is created in our minds, imagining the counterfactual, a world in which something entirely opposite and mutually exclusive occurs, is even more difficult. Our brains do everything they can to get around this kind of thinking. We naturally seem to prefer to use the parts of our brains that make rapid, intuitive judgments because this takes less effort than engaging the more evolved reasoning parts of the brain. Our limbic lobes fire before information even reaches the prefrontal cortex. If something is frightening, it stimulates another primitive part of the brain, the insula; if it is pleasurable and rewarding, it stimulates the nucleus accumbens, a part of the ventral striatum. The more noise, confusion, and emotion there is, the more likely that we will default to the amygdala, insula, and nucleus accumbens to make decisions based on impressions rather than probabilities. In order for us to suppress these brain systems and try to reason out a sensible decision based on data-based probabilities, we have to be calm, the environment has to be quiet, and we have to be approached by someone genuinely interested in our figuring out a solution rather than merely assenting to one.

Unless we devote the time and energy to assessing risk, we will default decision making to the impulsive brain, which makes statistical inference seem wildly counterintuitive, uncomfortable, unfamiliar, and generally strange and foreign. And this goes for experts as well as laypeople. In a famous experiment, 238 outpatients with different chronic medical problems, 491 graduate students at the Stanford Business School who had completed several courses in statistics and decision theory, and 424 physicians were asked to choose between radiation and surgery to treat a patient with lung cancer based on different sets of outcome probabilities.[27] Half of the subjects had the outcomes presented to them in terms of the probability of dying from each treatment (mortality risk) and the other half in terms of probability of living (survival chance). Strikingly, the participants who were told that there was a 68% chance of living for more than 1 year after surgery were most likely to choose surgery over radiation, but subjects who were told there was a 32% chance of dying 1 year after surgery were more likely to choose radiation. Perhaps even more surprising is the fact that the results did not differ by group. Physicians with experience in reading the medical literature and making intervention decisions and graduate students with expertise in statistical analysis succumbed to the same illusion as the patient group. That is, when confronted with the word *dying* everyone—even experts—ignored the data and made an emotional decision against surgery, but upon hearing the word *living* everyone chose exactly the opposite, even though there is in fact absolutely no difference in outcome between the mortality risk and chance of survival. The difference is only in how the outcome is worded or *framed*.

Even Experts Mess Up

Even professional statisticians can become lazy about probabilities and make easy judgments rather than engaging a slow, deliberate process of evaluation. In most medical studies the data are analyzed in such a way as to derive a probability value, or *p* value. You will see in the Results section of most of these papers a statement like "The difference between the two treatments was significant ($p < 0.05$)." If *p* is larger than 0.05, the difference is considered "not significant" and the study declared a failure. This convention has been accepted for over 100 years by scientists and statisticians alike, who often look only for the size of the *p* value to judge whether a study worked out or not. It took the mind of a brilliant and unusually charismatic statistician, Jacob Cohen, to point out the fallacy in such thinking.

A *p* value of 0.05 means that the probability that we found this result simply by chance is less than 5%. How was this level of significance decided upon? Basically, statisticians in the 1920s decided that it seemed about right to them. However, it turns out that the formula for calculating the *p* value is highly dependent on the number of subjects in the study. With only 10 subjects in a study in which half get Drug A and half Drug B, no matter how much better Drug A might be than Drug B the formula will usually not generate a *p* value of less than 0.05. On the other hand, if one could enroll 100,000 people in the study, then even if Drug A is just a tiny bit better than Drug B—a difference not even worth bothering with in real-life terms—the formula might generate a *p* value of less than 0.05. Jack Cohen had to point out over and over again that one cannot simply accept the *p* value as the entire basis for deciding if the outcome of a study is meaningful, yet to his ongoing chagrin most scientific journals ignored him and until the last few years relied exclusively on *p* values. So once again, an easy convention, one that requires little thought or effort, appeals to even the most brilliant statistician.

We Believe It if We Can See It

Numerous research studies have indicated a strong arsenal of heuristics and other strategies most people have formed to judge probabilities. A common heuristic is availability. The availability heuristic allows individuals to judge the probability of an event by the ease with which they can imagine that event or retrieve instances of it from memory. That is, if you grew up in Syracuse and you are asked about the likelihood of snow in October in the United States, your availability heuristic will cause you to estimate a higher probability than someone who grew up in Pennsylvania.[28] This heuristic is similar to Slovic's observation that dangerous situations that can be readily visualized and imagined are viewed as more likely to occur than situations that are not accompanied by readily formed mental images.

Similarly, a great deal of research has shown that we rely on stories and anecdotes rather than on statistics to judge representativeness and probability. Many of us can probably relate to this impulse or have witnessed it in our everyday lives. One of us (Sara) has a good recent anecdote illustrating this very point. After researching the concept of retail medical clinics and amassing a large amount of evidence that care under nurse practitioners for a wide array of common acute illnesses results in equally good health outcomes as care under a primary care physician, Sara found herself discussing the topic with a friend. The friend immediately interjected with a story about a time when he went to see a nurse practitioner for a case of bronchitis and the nurse practitioner did a poor job of diagnosing and treating the condition, resulting in a subsequent trip to the doctor and a longer period of illness. The friend was a highly educated individual with a very good grasp of the scientific process and of statistics who nonetheless insisted, based on this single personal experience, that nurse practitioners were vastly inferior to physicians. For a moment, Sara felt that all of her diligent research had been debunked. But then she realized: her friend's story is completely irrelevant. The point is that these kinds of events may occur, but the research has shown that so many nurse practitioners perform at such a high level that the future probability of any individual considering seeking help from a nurse practitioner to receive poor care is actually extremely low. Yet the power of the individual story and the salient memory of events that really happened to us almost always outweigh the power of projections about future events.

Our inherent desire to link *imaginability* with probability can lead us into something psychologists and behavioral economists call *conjunction bias*. Imagine the following scenario: you meet Linda, a 31-year-old single, bright woman who majored in philosophy, has always been concerned with issues of justice and discrimination, and participated in protests against the Iraq War. Which of the following would you think is more likely: (a) Linda is a bank teller, or (b) Linda is a bank teller and is active in the feminist movement? Or, to take another scenario, which do you think is more likely: (a) a nuclear war between the United States and Russia, or (b) a nuclear war between the United States and Russia in which both countries are drawn into conflict by other conflict-laden countries such as Iraq, Libya, Israel, or Pakistan?[29] Most people choose option (b) in both cases. However, the correct answer, from a statistical probability point of view, is (a) in both cases. This is because scenarios with more detail are always less likely to be true than scenarios with less detail. The likelihood that all of these factors will occur concurrently is lower than the likelihood of one factor on its own. Think of it this way: all members of the group of socially conscious bank tellers must be members of the group of all bank tellers, but the reverse is not the case. Hence, it is impossible to have a greater probability of being a socially conscious bank teller than of being a bank teller. In addition, the population base rate of bank tellers is higher than the population base rate of bank tellers who are also active in the feminist movement. This means that if you meet a random woman in the street, regardless of her personal characteristics, she is more likely to be a bank teller than to be a bank teller who is also a vegetarian, even if she is selling vegetables, talking to you about vegetables, or wearing a sign reading

"Vegetables are great!" The conjunction bias can, as Thomas Kida points out, lead to "costly and misguided decisions." Kida notes that the Pentagon itself has spent a great deal of time and money developing war plans based on "highly detailed, but extremely improbable, scenarios."[30] This is a bias that distorts the laws of probabilities that even people as smart as U.S. presidents cannot avoid.

Empathy Makes Us Human

There is thus a significant tension between the laws of statistical probability and the propensities of our minds. As discussed earlier, we have the tendency to favor stories, anecdotes, and information that we can process using our imaginations. That is, we are most comfortable with information to which we can attach some form of mental image or picture. Abstract concepts, nameless and faceless probabilities, and simple facts are of much less interest to us than stories and images. This kind of thought process allows us to develop an all-important emotional characteristic: empathy. In an entirely utilitarian society in which we made decisions solely on the basis of probabilistic projections of maximal benefits, we would not care about people who were of no material value to us. Biologists and anthropologists battle about whether any species other than humans have the capacity for empathy, and even if they do, it is very difficult to detect. Without reliance on a human connection and without an interest in individual stories, we would all be less likely to care about the old lady who has trouble crossing the street or even to function well and work together in groups. Yet when it comes to thinking about problems that really *are* dependent on statistical probabilities, such as the likelihood of adverse effects from eating genetically modified crops or the chance that a certain danger will truly materialize for us, we do need to pay more attention to the numbers than to the stories of individual people, and it becomes highly challenging for our brains to make this switch. Most individuals we know who smoke cigarettes actually never get lung cancer. So if we relied on individual stories we might recklessly conclude that smoking is perfectly safe. It is only by analyzing population statistics that we learn that the chances of developing lung cancer are about 25 times greater for a smoker than a nonsmoker. The very facility that we rely on in large part to be human and function appropriately in our social environments turns into a mental trap when it comes to interpreting statistics and probabilities.

This situation can have dire consequences in making healthcare decisions. Who would not like a doctor who declares "I regard every one of my patients as a unique individual and make a treatment plan based on her own special needs and circumstances"? We all want that doctor, the very model of empathic caring. But what happens when this physician is confronted with a 98-year-old woman with end-stage Alzheimer's disease who is refusing to eat? The woman has no memory left, no idea who she or anyone else is, and a total inability to perform even the most basic functions of life. From population statistics it is predicted that with the placement of a feeding tube and forced feeding she will live for 2 more months and without it for 8 more weeks. Very few people would subject this elderly woman to the pain of having a feeding tube put in her if they appreciated the futility of doing so, but perhaps our exceptional doctor will say, "I am not letting her starve to death—that is not how she would want to die." According to Kahneman, this is not unusual: "This is a common pattern: people who have information about an individual case rarely feel the need to know the statistics of the class to which the case belongs."[31]

All of this goes a long way in explaining why our risk perception is so flawed. And indeed, risk perception theory may go a long way in explaining why some parents still insist that vaccines cause disorders such as autism in the face of abundant evidence to the contrary. Research into risk perception indicates that vaccines are an excellent candidate for being perceived as high risk: man-made risks are much more frightening than natural risks; risks seem more threatening if their benefits are not immediately obvious, and the benefits of vaccines against diseases such as measles and mumps are not immediately obvious since the illnesses associated with these viruses—but not the viruses themselves—have largely been eliminated by vaccines; and a risk imposed by another body (the government in this case) will feel riskier than a voluntary risk.[32] Research has shown that risk perception forms a central component of health behavior.[33] This means that if parents view vaccines as high risk, they will often behave in accordance with these beliefs and choose not to vaccinate their children.

Imaginability of risk as a determiner for its perceived salience is also important here. It has often been noted that few modern parents have ever actually witnessed a case of measles or pertussis but, sadly, more and more people have contact with some of the illnesses for which vaccines are routinely blamed, such as autism. As a result, we might say that vaccines have become a victim of their own success. In 1999, Robert Chen designed a visual tool to help explain this phenomenon: the natural history of an immunization program (see figure 10).[34] The beginning of an immunization program is characterized by high morbidity and mortality from the disease in question and extreme widespread fear of said disease. When a vaccine to fight the disease is introduced, euphoria follows. People are more than willing to get themselves and their children immunized against the culprit that has caused so much death and suffering. This phase may last for a long while, as long as the memory of the horrors of the disease is still fresh. But as soon as this memory starts to fade, and a new generation of people who never had or saw the disease comes of age, fear of the disease likewise begins to abate.

What follows is a broad spectrum of responses to vaccination. Most people will still comply with government regulations and physicians' suggestions to get their children immunized. But a growing proportion of individuals will start to show resistance to a medical intervention they now find unnecessary and unnatural. Examples of

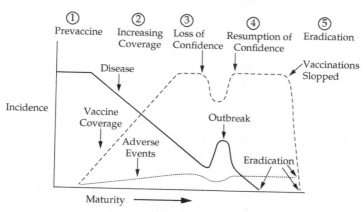

FIGURE 10 Natural history of an immunization program.

Source: M. Olpinski, "Anti-vaccination movement and parental refusals of immunization of children in USA," *Pediatria Polska*, 2012, 87(4), 381–385, figure 1.

disastrous effects of vaccines, however scant, will become exaggerated and widely circulated. The results of a recent nationally representative telephone survey demonstrate this principle well. In a survey of 1,600 U.S. parents of children younger than 6 years old, 25% believed that a child's immune system was weakened by vaccines, 23% believed that children get more immunizations than is good for their health, and 15% did not want their child to get at least one of the currently recommended vaccines.[35] In the absence of direct experience with diseases like measles and pertussis, parents believe that vaccines are unnecessary, that there are too many required vaccinations, and that their child's immune system would be better off without vaccines. In other words, they don't fear what they can't imagine.

The connection between the anti-vaccine movement and the psychological perception of risk described in this chapter is perhaps clearest in the favoring of stories over statistics. In fact, this feature is probably true of all of the health skeptics we describe in this book. The stories are there to remind us that the consequences of assuming a benefits-outweigh-the-risks attitude might be unbearable personal pain and loss. A good example of the reliance on personal stories comes from the ThinkTwice Global Vaccine Institute's website. The website's title makes it sound as though it represents an academic, evidence-based organization, but it is only a website and it is populated mostly by personal stories about alleged adverse reactions to vaccines. All of the stories are titled in large blue letters with the names of the children involved. The first story on the website reads:

> I recently took our only children, Harley (2 months) and Ashlee (2 years), to the doctor for their well-baby appointments. Harley had the sniffles and Ashlee had a cold, otherwise both were in perfect health. Harley was given his first DPT, polio, and Hib shots. Ashlee received her first Hib and MMR shots, as well as her third DPT and fourth polio shots. After the vaccinations I laid the children down for their naps. Harley woke first; his thighs were red. I heard Ashlee wake and then I heard a "THUMP!" Ashlee fell flat on the floor. She cried out "Mommy, me no walk!" I checked her over and stood her up; there was no strength in either leg. I called the hospital and rushed Ashlee to the emergency ward.... For ten days Harley's behavior changed. He barely slept, hardly ate, and seemed to be getting worse.

On May 17 at 9:00 a.m., my husband got up, checked on Harley, and yelled out, "Bonnie, get up, call the ambulance. Harley is dead!"

The use of these tragic stories illustrates the important connection between "imaginability" and risk perception. Once these stories are circulated, and especially when they proliferate, the newly produced ability to imagine an adverse reaction to a vaccine produces a sense of risk. In addition, we can probably all agree that it is more interesting for most people to read individual stories than to read the statistics about the probability of a child experiencing adverse effects as a result of a vaccine. What's more, we much more easily relate to and understand the story than the statistics. As we noted earlier, in many ways it is these stories, not the statistics, that make us feel human.

A Human Response

How can we mount a *human* response to a story like that of Harley and Ashlee that acknowledges the pain and suffering of the family who has lost a child but does not use it to sacrifice the value of vaccination? The problem here is partly due to the public's lack of scientific skepticism. After reading the prior quotation and recovering from the shock of graphically described tragedy, one might first ask if the story is even true. What turned out to be the actual cause of Harley's death? In a case like this, a postmortem examination, possibly including an autopsy, was almost certainly conducted. What did it show? Did Harley really die from effects of the vaccine? And if he did, as tragic as that outcome is, how common is such an event? In fact, it is extremely rare, whereas little children like Harley die on a regular basis from automobile accidents and gunshot wounds. All of this appeals to the prefrontal cortex rather than the amygdala and probably appears heartless. But how about telling a story about a 5-year-old with leukemia who is exposed to measles virus because of contact with an unvaccinated playmate? That child has a very high risk of dying because leukemia destroys immunity to viruses like the one that causes measles. Once again, we are left with the problem that public health officials are generally loath to "fight fire with fire" and use emotionally laden, manipulative messages to persuade us to do what the data show to be the right thing. Yet neuroscientists, psychologists, and behavioral economists document over and over again that emotional messages carry more valence than fact-based ones.

Why Buy a Lottery Ticket?

When it comes to vaccines, people also probably fall victim to a common misperception about the relationship between benefits and risks. Risk and benefit are usually positively correlated; that is, in most cases the greater the risk taken, the greater the benefit enjoyed. Skiers like to say things like "No spills, no thrills."

Research has established, however, that despite the fact that benefit and risk are most often positively correlated, they are negatively correlated in our minds. For most people, the greater the perceived benefit, the lower the perceived risk, and the lower the perceived benefit, the greater the perceived risk.[36] In the case of vaccines, the assumption promulgated by anti-vaxxers that vaccines are high risk means to some people that vaccines yield low benefits, because of this innate cognitive distortion.

In the case of the more recently introduced vaccine against the human papillomavirus (HPV), the virus that causes cervical cancer in women, anti-vaxxers had to go to great lengths to concoct a risk. It is claimed that the HPV vaccine will encourage adolescent girls to have sex. This claim is based on the notion that adolescent girls refrain from sexual intercourse because they are afraid of contracting HPV infection and getting cervical cancer later in life. By fabricating a risk that society abhors—young girls having sex—the anti-vaxxers not only scared some people but also took advantage of the risk perception distortion and created the myth that the vaccine must have little relative benefit. We have yet to see any evidence from even the most sloppily done survey that adolescent girls think that way or even how many have ever heard that HPV is the cause of cervical cancer. Now that the vaccine is available, there is no evidence that teenage sex has increased. There are, of course, convincing data that the rate of newly acquired HPV infection is already declining.[37]

Risk perception theory helps us understand in part why this assumption is so easy to make despite all the evidence from the past 50 years indicating that the benefits of vaccines are tremendous and nearly unparalleled in the history of medicine and public health. If we allow ourselves to believe for a moment that vaccines are very high risk, as anti-vaccination advocates insist, then it follows, based on the psychological processes that help us process risk information, that the benefits are miniscule. Alhakami and Slovic have characterized this process as an affective one. If an activity is "liked," people tend to judge its risks as low and its benefits as high. If an activity is "disliked," people tend to judge its risks as high and benefits as low. This affective assessment of risk has become second nature for most of us by the time we are old enough to decide whether to vaccinate our children. Therefore, if we decide that vaccines are high risk, it is difficult for anyone to convince us that their benefits are in fact high. On the other hand, when cell phones were said to increase the risk of brain tumors, there were no well-organized, vocal groups demanding their immediate withdrawal from the market. Some people opted to use earphones in order to keep the phones away from their heads, but there was no widespread anti–cell phone organization attacking the companies that make them or accusing the Federal Communications Commission of complicity. This is because people liked their cell phones and therefore were prepared to ignore any such risk. Some studies have shown there really is no such risk,[38] while others suggest that there may be some,[39] but in this case the actual level of risk appears to make little difference because we simply all want to use our cell phones.

We Are Endowed

Our perceptions of statistics are so prone to error and psychological adjustment that even the way in which a probability is framed can have a significant effect on how we interpret it. In addition, it turns out that our calculations about which risks to take are based much less on hard numbers and probabilities and much more on the ways in which these risks are framed. Behavioral economists such as Daniel Kahneman have discussed loss aversion extensively. The idea is that our psychologies teach us to be much more afraid of losing something than pleased to gain something of equal value. Kahneman and colleagues also refer to this as the "endowment effect." The idea is based on some experiments originating in the 1980s and 1990s that showed people's sometimes irrational desire to hold onto items they already owned, even if they were being offered better deals in exchange for them. In one simple study, participants were given either a lottery ticket or $2.00. Each subject was then later offered an opportunity to trade the lottery ticket for money or money for a lottery ticket. Very few subjects chose to take the experimenters up on this offer.[40]

Other, more complex experiments proved the theory of the "endowment effect" more solidly. In one experiment, 77 students at Simon Fraser University (SFU) were randomly assigned to three experimental conditions. One group, called the Sellers, were given SFU coffee mugs and were asked about their willingness to sell the mugs at prices ranging from $0.25 to $9.25. A second group, Buyers, were asked about their willingness to buy a mug in the same price range. A third group, Choosers, were not given a mug but were asked to choose between receiving a mug or the appropriate amount of money at each price level. The experimenters noted that the Sellers and Choosers were in identical situations, in that their roles were to decide between the mug and cash at each price level. In the end, the experimenters noted that the Choosers "behaved more like Buyers than like Sellers." The median prices were: Sellers, $7.12; Choosers, $3.12; Buyers, $2.87. The experiment effectively demonstrated that the resulting low volume of trade was more a result of owners' discomfort at parting with their endowment (e.g., the mug) than of buyers' reluctance to part with their cash.[41]

The endowment effect is reflected in brain function. Knutson and colleagues scanned research participants' brains with functional magnetic resonance imaging (fMRI) while they performed a buying, choosing, selling experiment similar to the one just described.[42] Activation was greatest in the nucleus accumbens—sometimes referred to as the brain's reward center—when contemplating preferred products across buy and sell conditions. Thus, whenever in a perceived favorable position, the brain registered a reward response. When, however, subjects were confronted with a low price for buying versus selling, a portion of the PFC was activated. Low price might seem attractive for a buyer, but it is also suspicious and activated a brain region dedicated to evaluating a situation carefully. Finally, during selling, greater activation of an adversity center in the brain, the insula, predicted stronger endowment effect: the stronger the activation of the insula, the more the emotional negativity at the prospect of parting with a current possession was experienced. Significantly, this last finding reminds us that individual differences are always greatly important in determining the results of both cognitive neuroscience experiments and real-world decisions. Some people are more prone to the endowment effect than others, for reasons that are as of yet not entirely clear but undoubtedly have to do with a combination of genetic endowment and life experience. It is not hard to imagine the evolutionary advantage of holding onto things one already possesses.

Clearly, the human brain is wired to promote the endowment effect, albeit with interindividual variation. Once we have decided that nuclear power, ECT, and GMOs are dangerous, we regard those attitudes as *possessions* and resist relinquishing them even in the face of a better offer—that is, even when we are shown data that contradict our beliefs. We have again another example of the way in which brain networks support a practical functionality that works less well when decisions involving complicated scientific issues are required.

Manipulating Our Moods

Kahneman and colleagues have noted that economic models that ignore loss aversion and the endowment effect credit us with much more stability and predictability than our choices actually reveal.[43] In the end, what these phenomena teach us is not only that psychology plays an enormous role in any kind of decision making, no matter how "rational," but also that in order to understand human decision making, especially surrounding risk, we need to take people's situations at the time of the decision into account. That is, the context of the decision matters and can help us understand some of the individual differences that exist among people's judgments about what is truly risky and what is not. A person's emotional state at the time of learning something new has important implications for how the content is processed and recalled. For example, as Norbert Schwarz points out, we are more likely to recall a positive memory when we are happy and a negative memory when we are sad or depressed.[44]

So, for example, let us imagine that the first time we read an article claiming that drinking unpasteurized milk will make our children strong and healthy there is an accompanying picture of a smiling, robust-appearing baby. Because this picture will make most of us feel happy, we will most easily recall the "fact" about unpasteurized milk when we are again in a happy mood. Similarly, suppose that when we first encounter the claim that withholding antibiotics from a person who has had a cold for more than 10 days is denying them good care there is an accompanying image of someone suffering with a nasty upper respiratory infection, complete with runny nose, red eyes, and distressed facial expression. That image will make us feel sad or unhappy and we will most readily recall the misinformation about antibiotics for colds when we are again in a bad mood. That is, the quality of the mood we are in when we first encounter a claim, regardless of whether it is true or untrue, becomes indelibly associated with the claim. We will associate consuming unpasteurized dairy products with happiness and withholding antibiotics for colds with sadness. Shrewd partisans of any cause understand this and therefore make sure to carefully manipulate our emotions when they present their ideas to us. That way, it is easier for them later on to get us into the desired mood when they present those ideas or conversely to make us recall the ideas with conviction when they once again rev up our emotions in a specific direction.

Experiments show that anxious people, as Schwarz goes on to explain, "pursued a goal of uncertainty reduction and preferred low-risk/low-reward options over any other combination."[45] If someone wants to make us afraid of genetically modified foods, their favored strategy is first to make us nervous about getting cancer and then tell us that the safest thing is just not to eat them, the lowest risk situation possible according to this view. Scientists, of course, prefer dry, factual expositions that are not intended to make people happy, sad, or anxious. While this is probably the most ethical approach, it also puts them at a distinct disadvantage to proponents of misinformation who may have no qualms about emotional manipulation. Recently, television advertisements aimed at getting people to quit smoking have been particularly graphic, showing people with advanced emphysema gasping for air and expressing heartbreaking remorse for having smoked. The ads may be effective, but some people decry them as inappropriate fear-mongering by the scientific community.

Several researchers have even thought about loss aversion in the context of people's reactions to policy changes. The most pertinent example is the public's attitudes toward the Affordable Care Act (ACA, also known as "Obamacare"). In the lead-up to the implementation of the ACA, investigators set up a survey experiment in an attempt to understand the relationship between loss aversion and attitudes toward various health plans. One half of the sample group was given the choice of the following two options: (a) a plan with no lifetime limit on benefits (chosen by 79.5% of respondents) and (b) a plan that limited the total amount of benefits in your lifetime to $1 million but saved you $1,000 per year (chosen by 20.5% of respondents). The second half of the sample group was given the choice between a different set of two options: (a) a plan that limited the total amount of benefits in your lifetime to $1 million (chosen by 44.2% of respondents) and (b) a plan with no lifetime limits on benefits but at a cost of an additional $1,000 per year (chosen by 55.8% of respondents). Both scenarios are effectively the same: the plan with no lifetime limits results in a loss of about $1,000, whether that is through not choosing the savings from the alternative plan or through a $1,000 cost directly tied to the plan with no lifetime limits. Yet nearly 80% of respondents in the first scenario chose the plan with no lifetime limits, while in the second scenario, this percentage dropped to about 56% when the $1,000 was explicitly framed as a cost associated with the plan with no lifetime limits. The idea here is that people are so opposed to the feeling of loss that they reject a scenario that they would have otherwise chosen if the $1,000 element were framed as savings rather than loss. Once again, the two scenarios are *identical*, but because they stimulate very different moods, they result in very different decisions.[46]

Not surprisingly, then, one of the public's greatest fears about Obama's healthcare reform was the prospect of *losing* something they already had: a particular doctor, a particular hospital, a particular health insurance plan. Wary of this, President Obama spent a lot of time emphasizing that the overhaul of the nation's health system would not result in any form of individual loss. In a 2009 speech to a joint session of Congress, the president emphasized this point:

> Here are the details that every American needs to know about this plan. First, if you are among the hundreds of millions of Americans who already have health insurance through your job, or Medicare, or Medicaid, or the VA, nothing in this plan will require you or your

employer to change the coverage or the doctor you have. Let me repeat this: Nothing in our plan requires you to change what you have.[47]

Perhaps without even knowing it, Obama was trying to get around a psychological mechanism that plays a significant role in our decisions and in our perceptions of much of the policy that surrounds us.

In an experiment published in 2010, Roger Bartels and colleagues at the University of Minnesota showed that framing is critical in convincing people to get vaccinated.[48] They designed their experiment in accordance with previous findings that gain-framed messages are most effective to promote health behaviors with minimal risk and loss-framed messages are most effective for health behaviors associated with more risk or with uncertainty. Undergraduates in psychology classes at the university were randomized to receive information that a vaccine for West Nile virus was either 90% effective or 60% effective in preventing disease and also randomized to receive either a gain-framed or loss-framed (this variation is noted in brackets) message as follows:

> By [not] getting vaccinated, people will be [un]able to take advantage of a way to protect themselves from a potentially deadly infection. If you are [fail to get] vaccinated against the virus, you can be [will not be] confident that you have given yourself the best chance to decrease your risk of developing serious complications from infection. . . . People who are [not] vaccinated will be free of worry [continue to worry] about mosquitoes and will [not] have the peace of mind to maintain their lifestyle.

This design results, then, in four separate groups of participants. They found that when the vaccine was said to be 90% effective, subjects who got the gain-framed message were more favorable to the idea of getting vaccinated, but when the vaccine was said to be only 60% effective, the loss-framed message was more effective. Clearly, simply manipulating how the very same information is framed has a profound impact on the decisions people make.

What does all this mean for our ability to perceive risks and make decisions about risks that affect our health? For one thing, there is a great deal of research to suggest that people are willing to take more risks in order to avoid loss. In health-related contexts, this means that people will react very differently to loss versus gain-framed messages and their corresponding willingness to take health-related risks will adjust accordingly. A loss-framed message in a health scenario might go something like this: in the context of preventive medical screenings for cancer, a doctor tells a patient: "If you don't detect cancer early, you narrow your options for treatment." This is a loss-framed message because the doctor emphasizes what will be lost by not taking the action of going through the screening process. This is like the idea that choosing the lifetime limit option on insurance will incur a loss of $1,000 as opposed to the idea that choosing the alternative plan will lead to a savings of $1,000. A gain-framed message about preventive behaviors might be: "Eating a lot of vegetables will help you become healthier."[49] In this case, the individual has been told that engaging in healthy, preventive behaviors will help him or her gain something: better health. Research has indicated that people view disease-detecting mechanisms, such as cancer screenings and HIV tests, as far riskier than disease-preventing behaviors, such as wearing sunscreen and taking vitamins. This is because disease-detecting behaviors have the capacity to reveal something disturbing, such as the presence of a malignant growth. Because people are willing to take more risks to avoid loss, it makes sense to use loss-framed messaging when trying to get people to agree to disease-detecting behavior. On the other hand, because people already view disease-preventing behaviors as low risk, it is much more prudent to use gain-framed messaging in these instances.[50]

The psychological mechanisms that interpret loss and gain differently clearly have an effect on risk decisions in health contexts. It would be wise for physicians and public health officials to familiarize themselves with some of these psychological mechanisms to better understand how to influence people to make the healthiest decisions possible. For instance, perhaps because getting vaccinated is a disease-preventing behavior, it would be more suitable to frame the need for vaccination to parents in terms of the benefits of health the child will enjoy rather than from the perspective of the diseases the child may contract if he or she is not vaccinated. An experiment could even be devised to test this idea.

Group Risk Is Not the Same as Individual Risk

Since a lot of people who deny the accuracy of valid health-related data have formed large groups and communities, it is worthwhile to consider how group assessment of risk might differ from individual risk assessment. The person who joins an anti-vaccine group on Facebook and then tries to make a decision about whether or not to vaccinate her child confronts slightly different psychological forces impacting her assessment of the risk involved than someone who makes the decision by reading a book about childhood illnesses or by talking to her pediatrician. The woman who joins the Facebook page is involved in a group risk assessment, and there is reason to believe that group risk assessment differs in vital ways from individual assessment.

One of the earliest studies of group risk assessment dates from 1961. Investigators concluded from an experiment that individuals make riskier decisions when in groups than when alone. They found that while an individual might decide to allow a form of surgery when there was a 1% chance of death, people in groups might allow the surgery with up to a 50% chance of death.[51] One scholar coined this the "risky shift phenomenon," whereby the amount of risk tolerated by individuals increased when they joined groups. Yet not all studies were able to replicate this finding. In fact, a number of subsequent studies found just the opposite: groups made decisions that were *less* risky than individual decisions. In response, psychologists and risk theorists developed the concept of the group polarization phenomenon, which asserts that groups cause individuals to become more extreme in their decisions. If you are somewhat predisposed to make a risky decision but may be on the fence, joining a group would, in this model, cause you to make an even riskier decision than you were previously contemplating.[52]

In a complex experiment, Scherer and Cho helped resolve the difference by demonstrating an extremely strong association between strength and frequency of interaction among people and agreement about risk assessment.[53] If Jane says hello to Harry only once a week in passing at work, she is much less likely to have a high degree of agreement with him on what is risky and what is not than if she speaks to him for 30 minutes every day. Of course, Jane might seek out Harry for more conversation *because* they are highly similar in many ways, including the ways in which they think about and assess risk. Nevertheless, under conditions of frequent contact the group polarization phenomenon seems to prevail: Jane's interactions with Harry are likely to strengthen her preexisting beliefs about risk now that she is in a group rather than an individual setting. Harry's beliefs about risk will likewise be strengthened. Scherer and Cho's work adds evidence that the extent to which Jane and Harry's risk perceptions will strengthen and converge is linked to the amount of contact they have.

This is perhaps an even more important concept now than it was when Scherer and Cho published their findings. Social media and the Internet make group formation much easier than ever before. In addition, the intensity and frequency of contact among people has increased exponentially with the development of new technologies and the increasing use of quick communication channels such as text messaging, Facebook, and Twitter. Many social media sites feature "groups" that individuals can join. Once you join a group, you are instantaneously part of a conversation that moves quickly and updates frequently. A sense of frequency and intensity of contact results easily from these forms of communication. According to Scherer and Cho's findings, the convergence of our beliefs about risk is likely stronger once we join that "Are GMOs safe?" Facebook discussion group.

Research on group risk perception has also emphasized the importance of social and cultural factors in risk assessment. In arguing for what has been termed the "social amplification of risk," sociologists proposed that it is a mistake to view risk assessment as an individual activity.[54] Instead, risk assessment is inherently social and responds to existing social and cultural norms. This argument moved the conversation even further away from the technical concept of risk: a simple multiplication of the probability of events and the magnitude of their consequences.[55] Because of this recognition of the more complicated nature of risk assessment, especially the ways in which risk perception responds to social and cultural environments, Kasperson developed the following model of cognitive process to explain the decoding of risk signals:

1. The individual filters the signals, meaning that only a fraction of all incoming information is actually processed.
2. The individual decodes the signal, deciding what it means to him or her personally.
3. The individual uses cognitive heuristics of the sort we have described in this chapter and elsewhere in this book to process the risk information.
4. The individual interacts with his or her cultural and peer groups to interpret and validate signals.

5. The individual and his or her groups formulate behavioral strategies either to tolerate the risk or take action to avoid it or react against the entities producing the risk.

6. The individual engages in actions formulated to accept, ignore, tolerate, or alter the perceived risk.[56]

Clearly this process is much more complex than simply multiplying the probability of the risk by the magnitude of its consequences and reacting accordingly. This account of risk assessment is also more complex than any model that asserts that information is received, cognitive heuristics are used to process it, and action (or no action) is taken. It incorporates a highly intricate social process into the perception of risk. Individual risk assessments are checked against group assessments, and action taken in response to these risks is both formulated and carried out in these same complex social environments. The idea that an individual assesses risk alone within the confines of his or her individual psychology, even though a more complex view than the idea that risk should be seen as probability times magnitude, is still too simple.

A quick look at a few websites can demonstrate how anti-vaccine advocates formulate strong group memberships that can shape people's perceptions of risks through the group processes described earlier. One website, VacTruth.com, "liked" by 48,514 people on Facebook, uses the term "vaccine pushers" to conglomerate "enemy" entities into one group, in response to which the identity of VacTruth. com followers becomes more concrete. Countless headlines on the site's "news" section use this phrase: "GBS [Guillain-Barré syndrome] Is Not Rare After Vaccinations: Here's How Vaccine Pushers Conceal the Truth," or "Bombshell TV Show About HPV Vaccines Reveals Cruel Nature of Vaccine Pushers."[57] The authors of the website effectively collect a series of anti-vaxxers' "enemies" into one group: pharmaceutical companies, the CDC, scientists at universities, the FDA, and other government agencies and organizations that promote vaccines. This simple phrase "vaccine pushers" creates a sense of a unified enemy around which the group identity of the anti-vaxxers can grow stronger. If we believe Kasperson's theory that group identities have a strong impact on both the formulation of risk assessment as well as action taken in response to these perceptions of risk, then we can see that the anti-vaxxers' strategy of strong group formation is a powerful one indeed and one that has the capacity to create people's sense of the risks associated with vaccines, regardless of what kind of statistical information organizations such as the CDC try to throw at them.

Another site, "VaccinationDebate," is much more explicit about the way in which it categorizes "us" versus "them." The author of the website explains why there is "misinformation" about the safety of vaccines:

> Firstly, they have you believe that there are all these germs out there that can kill you. Or if they don't kill you, they can cause horrible complications and long term suffering. Secondly, they have you believe that no matter how healthy you are, if you contract one of these germs then you can easily develop the disease and die. In other words, they have you believe that health is no protection. Thirdly, they have you believe that your only means of protection, your only chances of survival, is through their drugs and vaccines that you have to buy. (Your taxes are paying for them.)[58]

It is not immediately clear who "they" are, but if we think about it for a minute, it seems that the "they" here are the same as the "they" created by the VacTruth website described earlier. In other words, "they" are the CDC, the FDA, the government more generally, pharmaceutical companies, physician organizations, and medical researchers, all rolled up into one common entity. The "they" title again helps create a firmer sense of who "we" are and provides an opportunity for group risk assessment that goes something like this: the diseases vaccines supposedly protect us against are not risky, but the vaccines themselves present an unmitigated and potentially fatal risk. As discussed earlier, the presence of a group dynamic likely helps solidify this kind of assessment.

We have put this risk perception problem into a social framework to emphasize the importance of the community and social aspects in resistance to scientific information. But all of the weird principles of human risk perception still hold whether we look at individuals or groups. Our brains are not designed for linear risk perception even though that is how the world really is. Recognizing this is a crucial step in correcting our mistakes when we make health decisions and in planning interventions to help people make those decisions on a scientific basis.

Conclusion

W E HAVE ARGUED THROUGHOUT THIS BOOK THAT THERE are complex psychological, social, and neurobiological underpinnings of resistance to scientific evidence. We have also argued that many of these tendencies are in many ways completely adaptive, healthy, and essentially human. The challenge that remains for those of us interested in maximizing population health and at the same time helping individuals to make scientifically informed health choices is to figure out how to address the tendencies that lead to false scientific belief without completely insulting or, worse, attempting to repress these tendencies. Not only does telling people not to be emotional fail, but we also strongly believe that it is in no one's best interest to suppress this side of the human brain. So we propose a multipronged method to help guide people toward the evidence without dismissing the importance of their humanity. In the end, we don't want people to scramble for a story when they should be paying attention to statistics. But at the same time, we wouldn't want a society full of people who see only percentages and probabilities in place of showing empathy for the individuals around them. We just want to help people better tease out when their natural psychological tendencies are protecting them and when they are actually harming their health.

We will begin by citing the core principles that we believe any reader of this book should take from reading it. Then we will show how these core principles translate into our recommendations for better strategies for communicating and dealing with people who do not believe the science. We call this the Gorman-Gorman method.

Principles

Guiding Principle #1: It is not simply uneducated people who make irrational health decisions.

We have seen multiple times throughout this book that making rational health choices is not particularly correlated with intelligence. There are abundant examples of people with illustrious academic training, including in the sciences, who have embraced unrealistic and irrational beliefs about important topics such as the relationship between vaccines and autism and the cause of AIDS. The most prominent examples include people such as Andrew Wakefield and Peter Duesberg, both of whom had a great deal of scientific and medical training and illustrious scientific careers before building second careers espousing and proselytizing nonscientific and often dangerous ideas about health. It could not be argued that either of these individuals, along with many other examples like them, lack the ability to understand the science behind rational and irrational health choices, which is one of the prime factors that leads us to a more psychological approach to disbelief in scientific evidence. The problem is not ignorance but psychological forces that are in many ways surprisingly adaptive and important to human survival and the formation and endurance of human society.

We therefore strongly discourage any kind of approach to anti-vaccine, AIDS denialist, or any other nonscientific belief that revolves solely around assumptions of ignorance. Ignorance has clearly been shown not to be the prime factor in the formation of these nonscientific beliefs. Harping on ignorance, as many healthcare providers and public health officials do, will result only in further antagonism between the "scientists" and the "nonscientists" and will ultimately be unsuccessful in convincing a group of people who already understand the science to accept it. As we have shown throughout this book, the psychological and neurobiological factors driving these unscientific beliefs must be addressed first and foremost, not the educational level or scientific sophistication of the people who hold onto them. If combatting science denial were simply a matter of education our task would be far easier than it actually turns out to be, which brings us to our second point.

Guiding Principle #2: It isn't about a simple "lack of information."

There is a very strong tendency to attribute disbelief in scientific evidence to ignorance and a lack of information. In a *Forbes* article, Dr. Robert Pearl asserts that it is "important, especially for parents, to understand the potential consequences of preventable, infectious diseases."[1] A similar approach was taken in a 2001 article in *Vaccine*, as evidenced by the title: "Understanding Those Who Do Not Understand: A Brief Review of the Anti-vaccine Movement."[2] Both of these articles display a strong tendency toward the belief that science denialism has to do with a lack of information. As a result, a response of many public health officials and healthcare workers to health denialist beliefs has been to throw more information at "those who do not understand." Yet, as we have shown throughout this book, many people with denialist beliefs are highly educated and informational campaigns have tended to be unsuccessful. So we argue that simply throwing more data at people to prove that vaccines are not dangerous but that infectious diseases are will never be enough to truly address the problem. Part of the reason this approach will not work is because it completely ignores the psychological, emotional, and social instincts accompanying science denialism that we have outlined in this book and that prove to be quite important in fueling these beliefs.

Guiding Principle #3: Empathy and evolutionary benefits may sometimes be at odds with rational thinking.

This book has shown how, in many cases, the psychological forces that help us to be good members of society and even allow us to survive can sometimes be antithetical to the demands of rational thinking. We have shown how social situations, such as the sway of a charismatic leader and a strong desire to form groups that provide important social benefits, can sometimes cause us to set aside our rationality in favor of emotional appeals, desire for community, and strong leadership cues. When the same group that loves the Environmental Protection Agency (EPA) for imposing strict carbon emission standards on industries, which corporate America hates, also accuses the EPA of conspiring with industry when it does not list a pesticide as a carcinogen, we realize that the overriding factor is not lack of information. Such groups are usually consumed with information, including scientific information that they refuse to believe. Similarly, when environmental groups insist that global warming is occurring because a consensus of scientists say so but claim that the consensus of scientists who support the safety of GMOs or nuclear energy are misguided, the ability to understand facts is not the driving force. Rather, the need to belong to a group that maintains its identity no matter what facts are presented is the fuel for these contradictory beliefs. This need is characteristic of people from every race, income level, intellectual capacity, and country.

We have also seen how the very basis of a functioning human society and often what makes us human—empathy—can cause us to favor stories over statistics and misjudge scientific fact. What's more, we've seen how even our most basic survival instincts have caused us to formulate ways of thinking that are not always conducive to scientific rationality. For example, our most basic survival can sometimes depend on making quick inferences, instantaneously picking up cues in our environment and using heuristics to interpret them, thereby attributing causality with limited information. Yet, at the same time, all of these instincts can become traps when we are attempting to muddle through and make sense of complex scientific information. It is crucial to recognize that some of our most beneficial impulses and cognitive processes can also be the most damaging when it comes to understanding a complex system such as the scientific process. Without recognizing this, we run the risk of ignoring some of the most fundamental reasons for holding onto nonscientific beliefs: in many ways, the processes that cause them are the very mechanisms that help us survive and thrive in human society.

Guiding Principle #4: Hypothesis testing lends itself
to an inability to profess absolute certainty, and people
are uncomfortable with this.

How do scientists come to decide that *X* causes *Y*? In reality, the
way in which scientific studies are set up does not allow scientists to
ever *technically* make the claim that *X* causes *Y*. This is because of
hypothesis testing, the statistical procedure by which scientists can
decide if they have found a potentially meaningful result. In hypothesis testing, you begin with a *null hypothesis*, which is the hypothesis that shows you found nothing. As we have pointed out, if you
are doing an experiment to figure out if Drug A works better than
Drug B, your null hypothesis would be: "There is no statistically
significant difference between the efficacy of Drug A and Drug B."
Then you would formulate an alternative hypothesis: "There is a statistically significant difference between the efficacy of Drug A and
Drug B." (Notice that even in your alternative hypothesis, you make
no mention of whether Drug A or Drug B is better—you are simply
stating the possibility of a difference.) Then, you carry out the experiment. We use statistics to test the null and alternative hypotheses.
If you find a significant difference between Drug A and Drug B, you
will then reject the null hypothesis. But you can never "accept" the
alternative hypothesis. The *only* option is to reject or not reject the
null hypothesis. When you make the decision to reject or not reject
the null hypothesis, you also set up a *confidence interval*, usually of
95%, which means that you can say you would find this same result
95% of the time. Notice that there is no such thing as 100% in statistics. It would actually be incorrect for a statistician or a scientist to
say: "I am 100% certain that Drug A is better than Drug B."

So where does all this leave us? The rules of science and statistics
force us to work within a framework of negation as well as only *near*
100% certainty. Students of epidemiology and biostatistics will tell
you that it can be very confusing to formulate the correct statements
after running statistical tests, and their professors *will* deduct points
from a test or problem set if they proclaim: "Drug A and Drug B
show statistically significant differences in efficacy. We can therefore
accept the alternative hypothesis." Such a comment would provoke
a well of red ink from the professor, who would likely chastise this
student, writing, "We cannot ever accept the alternative hypothesis.

We can only reject or not reject the null hypothesis." By the time these students have graduated and become scientists or statisticians themselves, they will therefore have "We cannot ever simply accept the alternative hypothesis" so drilled into their heads that they will never be willing to make that mistake again and will always be very careful about how they phrase their experiment results when discussing them with the media. This is why a scientist will never say something like: "I can tell you, with 100% certainty, that A does not cause B." Instead, they will say something like: "There is no evidence that higher levels of A are associated with higher levels of B" or "Drug B does not display the same performance as Drug A in clinical trials to date." This can be extremely frustrating. Our psychological forces prime us to look for certainty and reassurance. We just want to hear: "I can assure you that Drug B is better than Drug A." But a scientist will most likely not feel comfortable making such a categorical statement for fear of misrepresenting the evidence that the scientific method is actually set up to collect. Indeed, when "experts" like the ever-popular Dr. Oz do seem to go too far with the surety of their statements, they generally get widespread criticism from their peers. Thus there is a fundamental disconnect between the kind of evidence that reassures human beings and the kind of evidence that the laws of statistics and science allow us to collect.

There is a joke among epidemiologists that encapsulates this disconnect: the marriage vow between two epidemiologists goes "I promise to always fail to reject you." There is a reason why this is funny (to at least some of us). Imagine if we approached wedding vows the way we approach hypothesis testing. We would be forced to make statements such as this one, which are not very reassuring to the emotional needs of two people trying to establish a lifetime of devotion to each other. So instead, in our emotional and social realms, we make much more dramatically declarative statements, such as "I promise to always accept you, no matter what." This is the kind of statement that makes epidemiologists squirm. The problem is that we cannot simply turn off our emotional and social proclivities when it comes to scientific evidence. So when a scientist says "There is no evidence to date that guns in the home are protective," we are much more frustrated than if we heard "I can tell you with 100% certainty that guns in the home are definitely dangers and never offer any benefits." The scientist does not make the former statement because he or she really believes there is a chance that guns are safe; the scientist is simply reflecting the statements that *can* be made from the way in which scientific evidence is collected. Although ultimately the two statements are the same, we *feel* less reassured by the former than by the latter.

Guiding Principle #5: People respond more to emotion than statistics, but charismatic leaders use emotion and scientists use statistics.

As we have observed many times throughout this book, people respond more to emotional anecdotes than to population-based statistics, and this is in part an adaptation that allows us to have empathy and thus form functional societies. This inclination has nothing to do with professional training: it is as strong in a scientist as in a novelist. The thought of helping our spouse, child, or best friend is easier to grasp than of saving the population of a city, state, or country. The problem arises when we think about how people get their scientific information and what kind of information is more likely to be accessible and persuasive. When a doctor, late in the day, sees a patient who has had acute bronchitis for the last week, her focus is on the patient, not on the population. An antibiotic will probably not help the patient, but it also probably won't do the patient any harm. The fact that such needless administration of antibiotics causes antibiotic-resistant bacteria to flourish, jeopardizing the health of people in ICUs, is much more easily ignored.

We argued in chapter 2 that charismatic leaders are in part so successful because they appeal to people's emotions. In fact, this is an important part of being a good leader in general: appealing to people's emotional side can be more effective when trying to boost productivity than stimulating merely their rational side, and the two attitudes can even work at cross-purposes. Charismatic leaders are emotional leaders par excellence and do an outstanding job at making people feel special, included, and unified. This kind of leadership strengthens beliefs, no matter what they are. And this kind of group formation is such a basic human instinct that we felt we would be remiss to write an entire book about individual belief formation without paying some attention to group belief formation.

Yet when it comes to science, this kind of leadership is rarely helpful, and indeed it has revealed itself to be quite harmful in many instances. One only has to think about Thabo Mbeki, charismatic leader of South Africa, whose idea that HIV does not cause AIDS strengthened a devastating epidemic in South Africa that is still not under control today. Part of the problem is that the scientific community has not responded in kind to the efforts of anti-science charismatic leaders. As a result, we find ourselves caught between appealing, charismatic leaders telling us that vaccines and nuclear power are dangerous and guns and unpasteurized milk are safe on one side and dry, academic scientists on the other side citing *p* values and saying things like, "There is no good evidence to confirm the hypothesis that vaccines are associated with autism." Given our natural tendency toward emotion and the way in which emotional appeals motivate us, who are we more likely to listen to in this scenario? You don't have to be a conspiracy theorist or member of a cult to agree that you'd rather listen to Winston Churchill give a rousing, inspiring speech than sit through a statistician's appraisal of all of the studies on the link between HIV and AIDS. The former is a charismatic leader; the latter is not. It is nothing to be ashamed of: the way in which traditional science is presented to the public is often very boring. But if we are going to make a dent in the way in which scientific beliefs are developed, we are going to have to find a better way to form groups around confirming the scientific evidence and selecting scientifically credible charismatic leaders to lead them.

Guiding Principle #6: People have trouble changing their minds.

It turns out that we are extremely resistant to changing our minds. We are reluctant to unlearn lessons we've learned and integrated. When we are confronted with information that conflicts with what we already believe, we experience *cognitive dissonance*. Cognitive dissonance is extremely uncomfortable, and we do everything we can to dispel it. This is how people convince themselves that smoking is safe, that they do not need to eat vegetables, and that repeatedly skipping trips to the gym will not make a difference in their weight and health. We set up beliefs that suit us, and then our brains work very hard to make sure we can resist anything that seems to challenge these beliefs. Studies have shown that the power of this fight against cognitive dissonance is so strong that it manifests itself in predictable changes in regional brain activation, even among people who have supposedly changed their minds.

Indeed, some clear patterns from imaging studies emerge that help us understand why cognitive dissonance occurs. For example, if we initially get a feeling of reward from an idea, we will seek to replicate the feeling multiple times. Each time, the reward center in the brain, the ventral striatum and more specifically the nucleus accumbens located within it, is triggered, and eventually other parts of the instinctive brain learn to solidify the idea into a fixed one. If we try to change our minds, a fear center in the brain like the anterior insula warns us that danger is imminent. The powerful dorsolateral prefrontal cortex can override these more primitive brain centers and assert reason and logic, but it is slow to act and requires a great deal of determination and effort to do so. Hence, it is fundamentally unnatural and uncomfortable to change our minds, and this is reflected in the way our brains work.

So what happens when we are confronted with a field that operates largely through the negation of old beliefs? As we have noted many times throughout this book, science operates mainly by disproving old evidence. As Sara's biostatistics professor used to say, "When you finish a study and you have found a statistically significant result, your next task is to present that finding to other scientists and say, 'I found something statistically significant; now it's your turn to try to make it go away.'" And this is exactly how scientific research works: we do everything we can to try to attack our statistically significant results to see if they can falter, and if we can't, we pass the results onto others to see if they can make them falter. Eventually, either the results can be replicated so many times that they become believable, or, more likely, conflicting results are subsequently found and people begin to change their minds. This is how science progresses: through repeated falsification of old beliefs. But what about the fact we just noted that changing our minds is among the most unnatural actions known to the human species? Obviously this creates a fundamental problem with our appraisal of scientific evidence. Science demands that we be open to changing our minds constantly, but human biology and psychology insist that we hold onto our beliefs with as much conviction as we possibly can. This conflict is fundamental to our reluctance to accept new scientific findings. Once the brain has set up the idea that GMOs cause cancer, it is basically impossible to undo that belief, no matter how many scientific studies provide evidence to the contrary.

Guiding Principle #7: People have trouble understanding probability and risk.

Decisions in medical science are predicated on the notion that we can determine a certain level of statistical risk and then use our judgment to apply that knowledge to specific cases. Medical decisions are therefore intrinsically based on a certain level of uncertainty, since statistical truth does not always translate into 100% reality for every individual. The fact that statistics can't always predict reality perfectly is extremely troubling for us, especially when it comes to making important decisions about our health.

Often, psychological forces therefore intervene between the statistical probabilities and how we use them to make decisions. A 1% chance of developing cancer means something very different than a 1% chance of developing a bacterial sinus infection. We are much more likely to take the former seriously, even to the point of accepting a series of treatments with serious side effects and high risks, and ignore the latter. The risk level is the same in both scenarios, but the decision we make is very different. Is it rational to pursue aggressive treatment for a 1% chance of something? Possibly not. We might act "rationally" when it comes to the sinus infection, but "rational" means less to us when it comes to a potentially life-threatening disease. In our minds, that 1% suddenly becomes a mental image of dying from cancer and regretting that we didn't decide to attack it early. In reality, a better way to think about the probability would be to imagine that we were 99% cancer-free and 1% cancerous. But from a human perspective, this kind of exercise is absolutely meaningless and displays a crucial failure of statistical evidence to translate into natural human cognition and decision-making processes. Emotion has a profound effect on how we judge a naked statistic.

This disconnect between natural human thought and the kind of thought required by statistical evidence is a serious problem when it comes to evaluating scientific evidence to make personal decisions. It is almost impossible for a mother or father to accept even a 0.001% chance of a seizure occurring after a vaccination when it comes to his or her own child. In the parent's mind, a 0.001% chance becomes a picture of the child having uncontrollable seizures. And as we have pointed out throughout this book, this vivid mental picture is not necessarily a bad thing in principle: it is part of what makes us able to empathize and to place great emphasis on the care and safety of our own children. The problem, once again, is that when it comes to medical decision making, statistics are often much more reliable than mental images and emotion.

So what should we do about all of these cognitive and emotional challenges that make it difficult for us to take scientific evidence into account when making personal health decisions? We cannot completely eliminate the role of emotion and empathy, nor would we want to do that. We can, however, learn to incorporate these emotional responses into appropriate strategies to handle poor medical decision making.

We will now turn to a series of these strategies. As is the case with this entire book, there are strategies here for many different constituencies, including scientists, nonscientists, journalists, and educators.

Solution #1: Science must deal with increased access to various types of information via the Internet.

When the recent erroneous article by Brian Hooker came out claiming that the CDC covered up information from a study that demonstrated that vaccines cause autism in African American children, the Internet was immediately filled with blog posts and articles insisting that we cannot trust the government and their lies and cover-ups. One of us (Sara) did a small spontaneous experiment: How many pages of Google results would it take to get to an article that explained the results from a more scientifically informed perspective? It took Sara 10 Google result pages to find an article by an actual trained scientist taking the results of this study into account and carefully delineating why the methods of the Hooker study rendered its conclusions invalid. But how many people are actually patient enough to click through 10 pages of a Google search? We already know that it is difficult for us to change our minds once we have formed an opinion. By the time you get to page 10 of Google results (if you get there), wouldn't you already have been persuaded by nine pages of strongly worded posts and articles trying to convince you, often with graphic pictures and heart-wrenching personal stories, that vaccines in fact cause autism and that this study by Brian Hooker, who has a PhD, shows nothing other than the government's shocking and horrifying decade-long cover-up of Andrew Wakefield's original "breakthrough"? Such messages invariably employ the principles of charismatic persuasion that we have already shown are incredibly effective. In addition, as we have seen with our analysis of risk perception, people are already prone to being skeptical of vaccines, unfamiliar man-made products whose mechanism of action is complex and counterintuitive. The mention of the word *vaccine* may trigger a response in the brain's fear centers, like the amygdala, because it carries with it associations of painful injections, infectious diseases, and dire warnings of complications like autism, a devastating illness that has deeply affected the lives of so many American parents and has a largely unknown cause. As we have also shown, people are not comfortable sitting with unknown causalities and tend to "fill in the gap." The advice of the charismatic leader is rewarding—it tells us there is a solution to our fear: Don't vaccinate—that carries with it all the privileges of joining a group of passionate people. The nucleus accumbens is activated, and soon the words of the charismatic leader become reified in our minds, a kind of habitual thinking.

All of these factors, all very natural human responses, conspire against the poor scientist who has slaved away to write a thoughtful article showing the scientific invalidity of the paper causing all of this commotion in the first place. That beleaguered scientist, appealing as he is to the sluggish prefrontal cortex, does not stand a chance against the barrage of nine pages of conspiracy-theory-laden articles preceding his analysis. So what can she do to make sure her work is not for naught and that her important analysis can see the light of day and influence these crucial, often life-or-death, health decisions?

We propose that scientists not only become fluent in the kind of information we confront on the Internet but also that they join the conversation in a much more active way. We think that scientific and medical societies in particular have much to gain from formalizing a broad, far-reaching online and social media strategy. Yes, all scientific and medical societies these days have websites and send out e-newsletters and digitize their journals. But how many of them have a truly active Twitter or Facebook account providing up-to-the-minute coverage for the general public about important scientific and medical issues? We would venture to say very few. (See figure 11.) A good model to follow is that of the American Geophysical Union. It has over 20,000 followers on Twitter, and at the recent AGU meeting in San Francisco, staff and scientists live-tweeted from the conference as new information was being presented.[3] Incidentally, a large number of these Twitter followers are not scientists. In addition, they have 11 individual blogs that incorporate recent groundbreaking science into user-friendly articles.

Just as important, scientific and medical societies and government health agencies like the CDC, FDA, and NIH must learn to anticipate public fears and concerns and take action before incorrect ideas become unchangeable. The CDC should have reacted immediately to reports of Ebola outbreaks in Africa to reassure Americans at the same time as it urged us to devote resources to help Africans. Hooker's article should never have seen the light of day, but since it did, the CDC should have responded online immediately. While this approach in no way comes close to dealing with the problem of irrational health beliefs on its own, it may be a crucial step in the right direction and a critical part of a wider strategy. Scientific and medical societies might need to hire new staff for this effort, but in the end, it could actually be part of a movement that saves a lot of lives. So the next time Hooker or one of his associates publishes an article on vaccines and autism and people google "Hooker vaccines autism," one of the first things that should pop up is a blog post from the American Academy of Pediatrics briefly and accurately discussing why the article's methods produced spurious results and invalidated

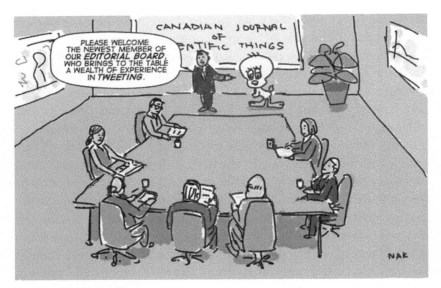

FIGURE 11 Tweet Expert

Source: "Tweet Expert," by Raymond K. Nakamura, 2013. Used with permission of the artist.

its conclusions. We know that this method will not prevent people who already believe that vaccines cause autism from continuing to believe that. However, efforts like this could prevent a large number of people who are confused or on the fence from being led down a path to dangerous medical decisions.

Solution #2: Members of the media need to be better trained to understand what a valid scientific debate is and what it is not.

There are obviously many legitimate debates in science, especially in medicine. Should the FDA speed up approvals of drugs for high-needs populations with severe untreatable medical problems? The answer to this is not straightforward: speak with two different doctors and you will get two different answers. On the one hand, it is essential to get people better treatment as quickly as possible. On the other hand, we need to be absolutely sure that the drugs we release are safe. There is no clear-cut answer here. Who really benefits from gluten-free diets? What causes irritable bowel syndrome?

What exactly is chronic fatigue syndrome, and who is at risk? All of these are legitimate questions up for debate in the medical and health fields. But other non-issues—such as whether vaccines cause autism, ECT is unsafe, or antibiotics treat viral illnesses—are not. The vaccine question was up for debate in 1998 when Andrew Wakefield first published his paper. But 17 years and numerous robust studies finding absolutely no association whatsoever later, this is not a legitimate debate among respectable and well-informed medical experts and scientists. How many more scientifically sound studies must be done before we have enough evidence to convince nonscientists what scientists already know—that GMOs don't harm *people*, just weeds and bugs. However, to an untrained person, these "debates" might look just as legitimate as the ones over the cause of irritable bowel syndrome, even though they are not. How should a journalist, who is usually not a trained scientist, be expected to detect the difference between legitimate and illegitimate scientific debate when the stakes seem so high in either case and, as we have shown, both types of debate involve preeminent scientists and medical figures?

We propose that all journalists who undertake scientific reporting, even if they have a PhD in a scientific field, should receive some form of training on telling the difference between legitimate and illegitimate scientific debate. The media must learn that the scientific method is not a variety of political discourse in which equal time must be given to both sides. The amount of time devoted to a side should be proportionate to the strength of its scientific evidence and the proportion of legitimate scientists who endorse it. Given these criteria, newspapers and magazines have to stop presenting the aforementioned non-issues as controversial. Why not institute continuing science education for journalists, as is required for many other types of professionals? A course on this precise skill could be a requirement in any scientific writing or journalism program. Clearly not every science journalist will go through this training, but if we can get a good majority to do it, the journalistic response to scientific debate might be a bit more accurate. We all want our newspapers and other media to spend more time reporting science, but it must be done in a scientifically sound manner. We consumers of scientific journalism should insist on reading stories written only by reporters who have maintained their understanding of the issues by demonstrating on-going participation in educational activities.

Solution #3: Scientists must be more sensitive to difficulties in communicating causality, people's discomfort with uncertainty, and their own weaknesses.

Scientists and medical researchers tend to be very intelligent, insightful individuals with a great deal of knowledge about their subject area. There is no doubt that scientific breakthroughs in the health and medical arenas are largely due to the unique insights of a handful of exceptionally skilled and dogged people. But this kind of intelligence does not necessarily translate into an understanding of how information should be communicated to the rest of us. Scientists and medical experts are simply not trained to take human emotion into account when transmitting the results of their research. So much of the focus in scientific training is on writing scientific papers for peer-reviewed journals that are read by other experts. However, little, if any, attention is paid to how to translate research into information for general consumption. There is some talk in science about making the results of scientific studies understandable to nonscientists: not using scientific jargon, explaining what specialized terms mean, and so on. However, as we have shown throughout this book, the issue is not necessarily that people do not understand the information on a basic level; the issue is that they interpret it in the context of a series of psychological processes that can sometimes distort the real nature of the evidence. This is the aspect that scientists need to grasp much better. Medical and PhD training programs for researchers should include lectures and exercises involving this type of general communication of complex scientific results. Discussion should center on not only how to make the material accessible but also how to present it in a manner that will discourage irrational responses. This is particularly important in areas of great uncertainty or seemingly high risk. Instead of just telling people the percent risk, scientists need to understand what these percentages actually mean to people and, most important, frame them in a way that they will be most convincing and acceptable to the nonscientists. A small amount of training in cognitive psychology and behavioral economics should make scientists more aware of the biases and heuristics people use to interpret scientific information and teach them how to communicate around these psychological processes so that their messages can have maximum impact and be interpreted in the way they intend.

Scientific journal editors must always bear in mind the possibility that articles they accept for publication will emerge on the Internet and be seen—and misinterpreted—by nonscientists who are not the intended audience. An article reporting that a new drug caused tumors in cancer-susceptible rats only at extremely high doses is reassuring to experts in drug toxicology but may hit the Web as scary evidence of cancer-producing medications. From there it is only a short step to conspiracy theories about the government and drug industry colluding to protect toxic drugs. We do not at all mean that the journals should stop publishing such articles—they represent vital steps in getting new medications that we need. Rather, the journals involved must develop ways to explain the content of these articles to nonscientists before things get out of hand.

We have stressed that it is not known how best to communicate scientific evidence in all cases and that some research has yielded surprising results that confound what we thought should work. Hence, there is a critical need for funded research on the best ways to communicate scientific evidence and perceived scientific controversies. Prospective, randomized trials of different methods need to be done until we get a better feel for what works and what doesn't. Should scientists use scare tactics? Do we need our own coterie of charismatic leaders? How do we transmit facts in a way that appeals to our audience's emotional needs, not just their intellectual ones?

In addition to understanding the psychological processes that accompany consumption of health and medical information, scientists and medical researchers must be more open about the mistakes science has made in the past. If we defend science too strongly and never admit to any weaknesses, we will only further alienate the public. Scientists and medical researchers should be taught about the value of uncertainty—if people are made aware that there is some uncertainty in the information presented to them, they may be able to more closely evaluate their psychological responses. Openness about past errors shows a certain ability to be self-reflective and will bolster public trust in the scientific community. Whether we like it or not, many people greatly distrust the scientific and medical communities. Rather than writing these people off, scientists and medical experts need to couch their findings with a compassionate understanding of some of these fears and reservations. After all, some of these anxieties and doubts do come from serious missteps in scientific and medical history, such as the ethical breach represented by the infamous Tuskegee syphilis study, the stubborn persistence in advocating against fat intake, or the inadvertent dispensing, to approximately 260 children, of early batches of the new Salk polio vaccine that contained some inadequately deactivated virus particles (that problem was quickly recognized and remedied). Mistakes are going to happen, but they must not be used as weapons against the validity of the scientific method or to bolster conspiracy theories.

Solution #4: We need better childhood education about statistics and probability, in-depth understanding of the scientific method, places for error in science, development of critical thinking skills, and techniques to understand what's "good evidence."

One of your authors (Sara) will always remember a project her older sister was assigned for science class in sixth grade. Rachel had to walk around town, picking up a variety of leaves, taping them into a notebook, and somehow finding out what type of tree they fell from. Sara never forgets this because the project tortured Rachel. Every time the family went out, Rachel got very nervous about finding "good" leaves. Then when she got home, she proclaimed (rightfully) that she had no idea how to figure out what kind of leaf her dried out and crushed specimens were. Her parents (including the coauthor of this book) spent hours (fruitlessly) trying to help. We could ask Rachel today whether she remembers that project. She would say yes, she remembers the pain and agony she went through to finish it on time. But if we asked her whether she remembers what any of those leaves were? No way. On the other hand, Rachel ultimately majored in biology in college and today she is a physician and must use statistical information every day to make important medical decisions that will have a deep impact on people's lives and well-being. What if we asked Rachel when was the first time she learned anything substantial about statistics? It was probably toward the end of her time in college. Almost nothing about it was ever mentioned in medical school.

Physicians are by no means the only people who need a deeper understanding of statistics and risk prediction. We are all bombarded with statistics, many taken inappropriately out of context, every day. With the rise of the Internet, the deluge of data, and a movement toward "patient empowerment," the need for us to understand statistics in order to make our own crucial medical decisions becomes more urgent by the day. Most Americans, however, are woefully unprepared to do this. As a variety of open access journals proliferate, many patients and their caregivers are now going online to read scientific studies themselves. But are these patients and their families really prepared to evaluate the nuances of a case-control study versus a retrospective cohort study, the true meaning of an odds ratio, and whether the sample size was truly sufficient to draw any conclusions? Not likely. We are not advocating that every person in America become an expert statistician or epidemiologist. However, we do believe that introducing some of these concepts in a general way early and often could make an enormous difference in the way in which average Americans approach data.

Throughout this book we have outlined many of our ideas for how this would work. However, there are a few worth highlighting. Early education needs to do a better job of teaching critical thinking techniques. By that we mean teaching children when to question something and when something seems solid enough to trust. This seems like a simple matter, but we are generally extremely unprepared for the task. Teachers could develop projects that make better use of the Internet, for example. Students could be assigned a somewhat controversial topic with a lot of conflicting data. They could then be told to use the Internet to collect as much information as they can. They could be asked to decide what information seems valid and what does not and outline their process for coming to this conclusion. Then a class discussion could examine how we make these decisions. In fact, as we outline in chapter 5, there are some relatively simple rules of thumb for deciding whether information is valid. One straightforward way is based on the way the website looks. Professional websites, like the website of the American Academy of Pediatrics, usually look polished and refined, while the websites of anti-vaccine activists usually look flashy and frenetic. Teachers could give students some rules of thumb like this that they could add to their strategies for distinguishing good information from bad. Children of the next generation will need to be able to wade through more online information than children of any previous generation, so they will need this kind of education more than ever before.

Teachers, and science teachers in particular, need better education themselves. Right now, teachers are often unsure of themselves when dealing with science, especially if they perceive that a topic is "controversial." As Melissa McCartney recently advocated, teachers need to be taught how to think like scientists, not merely to learn scientific facts and educational techniques.[4]

Finally, we believe that there needs to be a change in the way the scientific method is taught. Today, if the scientific method is taught to children at all, it is presented as if it were an enshrined, no-fault process that helps scientists arrive at an unquestionable answer. This makes it hard for most of us to ever understand how it is possible for a scientific study to become invalid after repeated failures to replicate. Instead, students should be taught about the basic structure of the scientific method, but they should also have some exposure to the messiness of it all. Where exactly can things go wrong in a scientific study? Students should be actively exposed to examples of this and be asked to evaluate simplified versions of published studies. There is no need to wait until someone is an advanced graduate student to teach them the basics of study design, bias, confounding, and statistical error. At that point, we find ourselves in a situation of simply preaching to the choir, which creates an even greater rift between the scientists and the so-called scientifically illiterate. There is no need for this distinction to be so stark, and we believe that the best way to address it is to do it as early and as often as possible.

Solution #5: We need healthcare professionals who can engage in motivational interviewing with people who have incorrect medical beliefs.

Motivation interviewing (MI) focuses on first finding out what someone knows and cares about rather than trying to convince them about something. It has been used very successfully in areas like addiction treatment. Addicts are often initially unwilling to change their behavior. A traditional approach is to inform them about all the risks and dangers of using illicit drugs and tell them they have to stop. The approach meets with very little long-term success. MI, on the other hand, starts by asking the addict if there are things in his life that aren't going well, that he would like to change. An addict may not be eager to give up the feeling he gets from snorting cocaine, but is unhappy with getting arrested or spending every paycheck buying drugs. Through this kind of inquiry, the interviewer finds common ground that becomes the basis for motivating the addict to change his drug use.

We believe this approach may also work when dealing with people with fixed but incorrect scientific ideas. Rather than telling someone straight out that vaccines are safe and effective and she should immunize her children, it may work better to begin by finding out the basis for her beliefs. What does she think, and how did she reach these conclusions? Along with this, the interviewer will find out what is important to this parent, presumably ensuring the safety of her children but also not jeopardizing the health of other children. A Socratic dialogue is developed in which the interviewer and parent share information and values to reach a joint decision. That decision may at first be simply to have another conversation in a week. Part of our research agenda is to test the ability of MI to successfully change health decision behaviors in a more scientific direction and to see if population-based MI techniques might be developed to reach larger numbers of people.

Solution #6: We all must examine our tendency to think uncritically and to place emotion over reason.

Poets, ethicists, and clerics have long lectured to us that the most exalted human state is love for and from another individual. We do not dispute this. But science can rarely afford to be sentimental given its responsibility to learn about the big picture, what will help the greatest number of people. To be a participant in this process, we are asked to set aside some basic biological processes that have been entrenched by millennia of evolution and to place reason over human instinct. This is not easy. Too much reason and we will never drive a car again and perhaps stop eating and breathing altogether since there seems to be a study somewhere, reported to us with glaring headlines, that almost everything we eat and breathe is bad for us. A life full of love, spontaneity, and enjoyment requires obeisance to emotions and heuristics.

As we have tried to make clear, however, the scientific process is rarely spontaneous or straightforward. It is full of fits and starts, rethinking what was once considered proven, and battling over what constitutes enough evidence to prove truth. It is so easy for us to be swayed away from the complexities and uncertainties of science by charged, graphic, and emotional appeals. We are not to be blamed for believing that anything made by a large, for-profit company must be evil, that medical associations say things only because they want to maintain their power over us, and that there are no government agencies that can be trusted. The facts, however, are not so simple. Drug companies do some awful things, but they also produce the life-saving medications that have revolutionized the prospects for human health and survival. Big companies try to sell us dangerous products all the time, but sometimes, as in the case of GMOs and nuclear power, they have hit upon technologies that, while not perfect, are far less risky and far more beneficial than detractors would have us believe. "Farm to table" and "back to nature" are wonderful ideas, often providing us with very delicious things to eat, but the "unnatural" process of pasteurization is critical to ensuring we do not get infected with life-threatening bacteria.

The only way that we can figure out what to believe is to school ourselves in the scientific method, to demand to know where people are getting their data from and with whom they are affiliated, and to reserve judgment until we have considered lots of points of view. Always ask "Compared to what?" and "What is in the rest of the boxes?" when someone makes a claim about the risk or safety about anything regarding our health. Above all, make learning about science an important part of your and your family's life.

A Final Word

Some people's views will never change. But if we can reach those people who are unsure and keep them from buying into incorrect scientific ideas, then we can declare a triumph. Undergirding our efforts to reach people should always be understanding and compassion. No one is immune from bias, heuristics, or emotional decision making. As we have hopefully made clear throughout this book, we are ready to admit our own foibles in these arenas, and this readiness certainly does not mean that we will not be prone to them over and over again. Even Daniel Kahneman admitted that he sometimes buys lottery tickets.[5] We know we cannot overcome the incredible power of emotional and social forces that sometimes lead us astray in our scientific thinking, nor do we want to do that. It is not our intention to promote a world in which people do not care about stories, do not come together over issues that bother them, and do not feel inspired by charismatic leaders. But we do want to emphasize that until we bring these psychological, emotional, and social forces into the conversation, we will never get anywhere in the struggle against dangerous, unscientific ideas. As we hope we have shown, the answer to the question we set out to solve, why people cling to irrational medical and health views with no scientific basis, is as simple as this: because we are human. We are humans with empathy and a strong drive to build communities. We would never advocate eroding these wonderful features of human nature.

So we need to take them fully into account when we plan strategies to improve our ability to grasp scientific reality. Vaccinate your children, understand the benefits and not just the risks of GMOs and nuclear power, don't drink unpasteurized milk or take antibiotics for a virus, agree to ECT if depression is overwhelming and refractory to drugs, and don't buy a gun. Every one of these recommendations will invoke powerful feelings, including rage, in many people, but every one of them is based on the overwhelming weight of scientific evidence. By adding compassion, empathy, and emotion into this equation we will finally be able to effectively help people make the crucial decisions that will ultimately save their lives.

Notes

Introduction

1. A. Mamiit, "Relatives of Thomas Eric Duncan blame Ebola victim's death on hospital's lack of proper care," *Tech Times*, October 12, 2014, http://www.techtimes.com/articles/17683/2141012; Manny Fernandez & Dave Philips, "Death of Thomas Eric Duncan in Dallas fuels alarm over Ebola," *The New York Times*, October 8, 2014; Alexandra Sifferlin, "Here's who's blaming who for Ebola," *TIME*, October 16, 2014, http://time.com/3513274/ebola-cdc-obama-blame/
2. D. Baker, "Ebola hysteria fever: A real epidemic," *Huffington Post*, October 21, 2014.
3. A. Yuhas, "Panic: The dangerous epidemic sweeping an Ebola-fearing US," *The Guardian*, October 20, 2014.
4. C. M. Blow, "The Ebola hysteria," *The New York Times*, October 29, 2014.
5. S. L. Murphy, J. Xu, K. D. Kochanek, United States Department of Health and Human Services, & Centers for Disease Control and Prevention, *National vital statistics reports, Deaths: Final data for 2010*, May 2013, 61. We have simply divided the total numbers of deaths for 2010, the most recent complete report

available, by 365. Of course, these numbers fluctuate for causes of death that are seasonal, such as influenza, but give a fairly good idea of the magnitude on a daily basis in the United States.

6. http://www.npr.org/blogs/goatsandsoda/2014/10/23/358349882/an-answer-for-americans-who-ask-whats-my-risk-of-catching-ebola, October 23, 2014.

7. B. Hallowell, "Pastor solves mystery surrounding why one-fourth of his congregation abruptly disappeared," *The Blaze*, June 6, 2015.

8. E. Ritz, "Nurse diagnosed with Ebola makes a request of Ohio bridal shop that the owner is calling a 'slap in the face,'" *The Blaze*, November 26, 2014.

9. "Report slams U.S. Ebola response and readiness," *NBCNews*, February 26, 2015.

10. http://blogs.plos.org/speakingofmedicine/2014/10/22/ebola-taught-us-crucial-lesson-views-irrational-health-behaviors/

11. C. Spencer, "Having and fighting Ebola—public health lessons from a clinician turned patient," *New England Journal of Medicine*, 2015, *372*, 1089–1091.

12. S. B. Omer, D. A. Salmon, W. A. Orenstein, P. deHart, & N. Halsey, "Vaccine refusal, mandatory immunization, and the risks of vaccine-preventable diseases," *New England Journal of Medicine*, 2009, *360*, 1981–1988.

13. A. Anglemyer, T. Horvath, & G. Rutherford, "The accessibility of firearms and risk for suicide and homicide victimization among household members: A systematic review and meta-analysis," *Annals of Internal Medicine*, 2014, *160*, 101–110.

14. N. Golgowski, "Woman kills self with gun bought for Ferguson unrest: Report," *New York Daily News*, November 24, 2014, http://www.nydailynews.com/news/national/woman-kills-gun-bought-ferguson-unrest-report-article-1.2022352

15. O. Khazan, "Wealthy LA schools vaccination rates are as low as South Sudan's," *The Atlantic*, September 16, 1951, http://www.theatlantic.com/health/archive/2014/09/wealthy-la-schools-vaccination-rates-are-as-low-as-south-sudans/380252/

16. C. Pouliot & J. Godbout, "Thinking outside the 'knowledge deficit' box," *EMBO Reports*, 2014, *15*, 833–835.

17. L. Xin, "Got charisma? Depends on your voice," http://news.sciencemag.org/biology/2014/10/got-charisma-depends-your-voice, October 29, 2014.

18. P. Slovic, "Beyond numbers: A broader perspective on risk perception and risk communication," in Deborah G. Mayo & Rachelle D. Hollander, eds., *Acceptable evidence: Science and values in risk management*, Oxford: Oxford University Press, 1991, 48–65.

19. D. H. Barlow, J. M. Gorman, M. K. Shear, & S. W. Woods, "Cognitive-behavioral therapy, imipramine, or their combination for panic disorder: A randomized controlled trial," *Journal of the American Medical Association*, 2000, *283*, 2529–2536.

20. By *body fluids* we mean saliva, mucus, vomit, feces, tears, breast milk, urine, and semen. One has to come into contact with one of these from an infected person or the corpse of someone who died from Ebola in order to get sick. Simply sitting next to someone with Ebola virus infection on a plane or bus is insufficient to catch it.

21. National Safety Council, *Injury facts, 2014 Edition*, Itasca, IL: Author, 2014.

22. D. Kahneman, personal communication.

23. N. N. Taleb, *Fooled by randomness: The hidden role of chance in life and in the markets*, New York: Random House, 2004.

24. http://minnesota.cbslocal.com/2014/10/06/widow-of-1st-american-ebola-victim-strives-to-end-ignorance/

25. http://www.cnn.com/2014/10/24/health/ebola-travel-policy/; Marc Santora, "Doctor in New York City is sick with Ebola," *The New York Times*, October 23, 2014; and finally, Anemona Hartocollis, "Craig Spencer, New York doctor with Ebola, will leave Bellevue Hospital," *The New York Times*, November 10, 2014.

26. C. Spencer, "Having and fighting Ebola—public health lessons from a clinician turned patient," *New England Journal of Medicine*, 2015, *372*, 1089–1091.

27. C. Spencer, "Having and fighting Ebola—public health lessons from a clinician turned patient," *New England Journal of Medicine*, 2015, *372*, 1090.

28. F. DeStefano, T. Karapurkar, W. W. Thompson, M. Yeargin-Allsopp, & C. Boyle, "Age at first measles-mumps-rubella vaccination in children with autism and school-matched control subjects: A population-based study in metropolitan Atlanta," *Pediatrics*, 2004, *113*, 259–266.

29. http://www.translationalneurodegeneration.com/content/3/1/22

30. B. Kantrowitz, "The science of learning," *Scientific American*, August 2014, 69–73; S. Freeman, S. L. Eddy, M. McDonough, M. K. Smith, N. Okoroafor, H. Jordt, & M. P. Wenderoth, "Active learning increases student performance in science, engineering, and mathematics," *Proceedings of the National Academy of Sciences (USA)*, 2014, *111*, 8410–8415.

31. A. Meisel, "Keeping science fun," September 2014, http://www.sas.upenn.edu/series/frontiers/keeping-science-fun

32. P. G. Alaimo, J. M. Langenhan, & I. T. Suydam, "Aligning the undergraduate organic laboratory experience with professional work: The centrality of reliable and meaningful data," *Journal of Chemic Education*, Epub October 10, 2014, doi:10.1021/ed400510b

33. R. Pérez-Peña, "Colleges reinvent classes to keep more students in science," *The New York Times*, December 26, 2014.

34. http://jeromiewilliams.com/2013/04/12/holy-fukushima-radiation-from-japan-is-already-killing-north-americans/

35. D. Kahan, D. Braman, & H. Jenkins-Smith, "Cultural cognition of scientific consensus," *Journal of Risk Research*, 2011, *14*, 147–174.

36. B. Nyhan, J. Reifler, S. Richey, & G. L. Freed, "Effective messages in vaccine promotion: A randomized trial," *Pediatrics*, 2014, *133*, e835–842.

37. J. K. Koh, "Graphic warnings for cigarette labels," *New England Journal of Medicine*, August 4, 2011, *365*, e10.

38. S. A. Schroeder, "Tobacco control in the wake of the 1998 master settlement agreement," *New England Journal of Medicine*, 2004, *350*, 293–301.

39. T. Nordhaus & M. Shellenberger, "Global warming scare tactics," *The New York Times*, April 8, 2014.

40. D. Shiffman, " 'I'm not a scientist' is a dangerous cop-out," http://www.slate.com/articles/health_and_science/science/2014/10/i_m_not_a_scientist_excuse_politicians_don_t_need_to_be_experts_to_make.html

41. A. Cockcroft, M. Masisi, L. Thabane, & N. Andersson, "Legislators learning to interpret evidence for policy," *Science*, 2014, *354*, 1244–1245.

42. C. Korownyk, M. R. Kolber, J. McCormack, et al., "Televised medical talk shows—what they recommend and the evidence to support their recommendations: A prospective observational study," *British Medical Journal*, 2014, *349*, g7346, doi:10.1136/bmj.g7346

43. G. A. Poland &R. M. Jacobson, "Understanding those who do not understand: A brief review of the anti-vaccine movement," *Vaccine*, 2001, *19*, 2440–2445.

44. G. K. Spurling, P. R. Mansfield, B. D. Montgomery, J. Lexchin, J. Doust, N. Othman, et al., "Information from pharmaceutical companies and the quality, quantity, and cost of physicians' prescribing: A systematic review," *PLoS Medicine*, 2010, *7*(10), e1000352, doi:10.1371/journal.pmed.1000352; B. T. Montague, A. H. Fortin 6th, & J. Rosenbaum, "A systematic review of curricula on relationships between residents and the pharmaceutical industry," *Medical Education*, March 2008, *42*(3), 301–308.

45. For a fuller discussion of these issues, see J. M. Gorman & P. E. Nathan, "Challenges to implementing evidence-based treatments," in Peter E. Nathan and Jack M. Gorman, eds., *A Guide to Treatments that Work*, 4th ed., New York: Oxford University Press, 2015, 1–21.

46. "Economists aren't free of biases, even though economists say otherwise," *The Daily Idea: Harvard Business Review*, September 16, 2014.

47. D. Martin, "Elizabeth Whelan, who challenged food laws, dies at 70," *The New York Times*, September 17, 2014.

48. To be fair, Whelan was almost certainly correct in challenging the notion that artificial sweeteners are human carcinogens. However, it is now clear that use of artificial sweeteners has the paradoxical effect of increasing the risk for type 2 diabetes.

Chapter 1

1. http://townhall.com/tipsheet/mattvespa/2015/03/03/nras-lapierreif-you-care-about-your-freedoms-you-belong-in-the-national-rifle-association-n1965197; https://www.nranews.com/series/wayne-lapierre/video/wayne-lapierre-how-to-stop-violent-crime/episode/wayne-lapierre-season-1-episode-1-how-to-stop-violent-crime; http://thinkprogress.

org/politics/2012/12/21/1368881/everything-you-need-to-know-about-the-nras-wayne-lapierre/; W. LaPierre, address at NRA-ILA Leadership Forum, April 25, 2014, https://www.youtube.com/watch?v=t3XJKAq8NjQ; W. LaPierre address to the 2014 Conservative Political Action Conference, February 6, 2014, http://dailycaller.com/2014/03/06/cpac-wayne-lapierres-speech/

2. C. Hodapp & A. Von Kannon, *Conspiracy theories and secret societies for dummies*, Hoboken, NJ: Wiley Publishing, 2008, 21. This volume was cited in another book by an author we consider both erudite and discriminating and were surprised to find that despite its title it has some useful information. We stress, however, that it is imperative *never* to use the word "dummy" or anything like it when referring to the victims of conspiracy theories. Such people are not at all unintelligent as a class and calling them so feeds right into the hands of the leaders of such groups.

3. U.S. Department of Health and Human Services, *The health consequences of smoking—50 years of progress: A report of the Surgeon General*, Atlanta, GA: U.S. Department of Health and Human Services, Centers for Disease Control and Prevention, National Center for Chronic Disease Prevention and Health Promotion, Office on Smoking and Health, 2014.

4. N. Oreskes & E. M. Conway, *Merchants of doubt: How a handful of scientists obscured the truth on issues from tobacco smoke to global warming*, New York: Bloomsbury Press, 2010, 6.

5. C. Mooney & S. Kirshenbaum, *Unscientific America: How scientific illiteracy threatens our future*, New York: Basic Books, 2009, 29.

6. It isn't, of course. The overwhelming scientific consensus based on extensive data is that climate change and global warming are real and alarming phenomena.

7. S. C. Kalichman, *Denying AIDS: Conspiracy theories, pseudoscience, and human tragedy*, New York: Copernicus/Springer, 2009, 9.

8. K. M. Douglas & R. M. Sutton, "Does it take one to know one? Endorsement of conspiracy theories is influenced by personal willingness to conspire," *British Journal of Social Psychology*, 2011, 50, 544–552, quotes on pp. 545 and 550.

9. J. A. Whitson & A. D. Galinsky, "Lacking control increases illusory pattern perception," *Science*, 2008, *322*, 115–117.

10. D. Jolley & K. M. Douglas, "The social consequences of conspiracism: Exposure to conspiracy theories decreases intentions to engage in politics and to reduce one's carbon footprint," *British Journal of Psychology*, 2014, *105*, 35–56.

11. V. Swamin, R. Coles, S. Stieger, J. Pietschnig, A. Furnham, S. Rehim, & M. Voracek, "Conspiracist ideation in Britain and Austria: Evidence of a monological belief system and associations between individual psychological differences and real-world and fictitious conspiracy theories," *British Journal of Psychology*, 2011, *102*, 443–463, quote on p. 452.

12. D. Jolley & K. M. Douglas, "The effects of anti-vaccine conspiracy theories on vaccination intentions," *PLoS ONE*, 2014, *9*, e89177.

13. S. Lewandowsky, K. Oberauer, & G. E. Gignac, "NASA fakes the moon landing—therefore, (climate) science is a hoax: An anatomy of the motivated rejection of science," *Psychological Science*, 2013, *24*, 622–633.

14. D. Jolley & K. M. Douglas, "The effects of anti-vaccine conspiracy theories on vaccination intentions," *PLoS ONE*, 2014, *9*, e89177, 6.

15. Jack freely acknowledges that this was once indeed his own thinking. Until a little over a decade ago he was the recipient of money from many drugs companies. Hence, this is not a statement generated from a false sense of moral superiority but rather from personal experience.

16. L. M. Bogart, G. Wagner, F. H. Galvan, & D. Banks, "Conspiracy beliefs about HIV are related to antiretroviral treatment nonadherence among African American men with HIV," *Journal of Acquired Immune Deficiency Syndrome*, 2010, *53*, 648–655.

17. M. Abalakina-Paap, W. G. Stephan, T. Craig, & W. L. Gregory, "Beliefs in conspiracies," *Political Psychology*, 1999, *20*, 637–647, quote on p. 637.

18. M. Bruder, P. Haffke , N. Neave, N. Nouripanah, & R. Imhoff, "Measuring individual differences in generic beliefs in conspiracy theories across cultures: Conspiracy Mentality Questionnaire," *Frontiers in Psychology*, 2013, *4*, 225.

19. T. Goertzel, "Conspiracy theories in science," *EMBO Reports*, 2010, *11*, 493–499, quote on p. 494.

20. A. Makrandya & P. Wilknson, "Electricity generation and health," *Lancet*, 2007, *370*, 979–990.

21. M. Gannon, "Air pollution linked to 1 in 8 deaths worldwide," http://www.livescience.com/44365-air-pollution-linked-to-1-in-8-deaths.html

22. D. Kahneman, *Thinking, fast and slow*, New York: Farrar, Straus and Giroux, 2011, 140.

23. A. Damascio, *Descartes' error: Emotion, reason, and the human brain*, New York: G. P. Putnam's Sons, 1994.

24. J. G. Edelson, Y. Dudai, R. J. Dolan, & T. Sharot, "Brain substrates of recovery from misleading influence," *Journal of Neuroscience*, 2014, *34*, 7744–7753.

25. P. Slovic, M. Finucane, E. Peters, & D. G. MacGregor, "The affect heuristic," in Thomas Gilovich, Dale W. Griffin, & Daniel Kahneman, eds., *Heuristics and biases: The psychology of intuitive judgment*, New York: Cambridge University Press, 2002, 401.

26. N. Schwarz, "Feelings as information: Moods influence judgments and processing strategies," in Thomas Gilovich, Dale W. Griffin, & Daniel Kahneman, eds., *Heuristics and biases: The psychology of intuitive judgment*, New York: Cambridge University Press, 2002, 535.

27. T. Goertzel, "Conspiracy theories in science," *EMBO Reports*, 2010, *11*, 493–499.

28. C. R. Sunstein, *Conspiracy theories and other dangerous ideas*, New York, Simon and Schuster, 2014, 5.

29. P. R. Bost, S. G. Prunier, & A. J. Piper, "Relations of familiarity with reasoning strategies in conspiracy beliefs," *Psychological Reports*, 2010, *107*, 593–602, quote on p. 599.

30. P. R. Bost & S. G. Prunier, "Rationality in conspiracy beliefs: The role of perceived motive," *Psychological Reports: Sociocultural Issues in Psychology*, 2013, *113*, 118–128.

31. P. R. Bost & S. G. Prunier, "Rationality in conspiracy beliefs: The role of perceived motive," *Psychological Reports: Sociocultural Issues in Psychology*, 2013, *113*, 118–128, quote on p. 125.

32. B. G. Southwell, *Social networks and popular understanding of science and health: Sharing disparities*, Baltimore, MD: The Johns Hopkins University Press, 2013, 8.

33. N. Hertz, *Eyes wide open: How to make smart decisions in a confusing world*, New York: HarperCollins, 2013, 169.

34. B. G. Southwell, *Social networks and popular understanding of science and health: Sharing disparities*, Baltimore, MD: The Johns Hopkins University Press, 2013, 72.

35. C. Mooney & S. Kirshenbaum, *Unscientific America: How scientific illiteracy threatens our future*, New York: Basic Books, 2009, 15.

36. C. R. Sunstein, *Conspiracy theories and other dangerous ideas*, New York: Simon and Schuster, 2014, 13.

37. V. Swami, "Social psychological origins of conspiracy theories: The case of the Jewish conspiracy theory in Malaysia," *Frontiers in Psychology*, 2012, 3, 280. Published online August 6, 2012. Prepublished online July 3, 2012, doi: 10.3389/fpsyg.2012.00280.

38. C. R. Sunstein, *Conspiracy theories and other dangerous ideas*, New York: Simon and Schuster, 2014, 22.

39. C. R. Sunstein, *Conspiracy theories and other dangerous ideas*, New York: Simon and Schuster, 2014, 29.

Chapter 2

1. S. A. Haslam, S. D. Reicher, & M. J. Platow, *The new psychology of leadership: Identity, influence, and power*, Hove, East Sussex, UK: Psychology Press, 2011, 29.

2. S. A. Haslam, S. D. Reicher, & M. J. Platow, *The new psychology of leadership: Identity, influence, and power*, Hove, East Sussex, UK: Psychology Press, 2011, 75.

3. S. A. Haslam, S. D. Reicher, & M. J. Platow, *The new psychology of leadership: Identity, influence, and power*, Hove, East Sussex, UK: Psychology Press, 2011, 75.

4. S. A. Haslam, S. D. Reicher, & M. J. Platow, *The new psychology of leadership: Identity, influence, and power*, Hove, East Sussex, UK: Psychology Press, 2011, 75.

5. J. A. Conger & R. N. Kanungo, *Charismatic leadership in organizations*, Thousand Oaks, CA: Sage, 1998, 23–24.

6. J. A. Conger & R. N. Kanungo, *Charismatic leadership in organizations*, Thousand Oaks, CA: Sage, 1998, 13–14.

7. J. A. Conger & R. N. Kanungo, *Charismatic leadership in organizations*, Thousand Oaks, CA: Sage, 1998, 15.

8. J. A. Conger & R. N. Kanungo, *Charismatic leadership in organizations*, Thousand Oaks, CA: Sage, 1998, 21.

9. R. H. Gass & J. S. Seiter, *Persuasion, social influence, and compliance gaining*, 4th ed., Boston: Allyn & Bacon, 2011, 121.

10. R. H. Gass & J. S. Seiter, *Persuasion, social influence, and compliance gaining*, 4th ed., Boston: Allyn & Bacon, 2011, 121–122.

11. http://www.psychologytoday.com/blog/spycatcher/201208/dangerous-cult-leaders

12. R. H. Gass & J. S. Seiter, *Persuasion, social influence, and compliance gaining*, 4th ed., Boston: Allyn & Bacon, 2011, 54.

13. R. H. Gass & J. S. Seiter, *Persuasion, social influence, and compliance gaining*, 4th ed., Boston: Allyn & Bacon, 2011, 62.

14. R. H. Gass & J. S. Seiter, *Persuasion, social influence, and compliance gaining*, 4th ed., Boston: Allyn & Bacon, 2011, 186.

15. J. A. Conger & R. N. Kanungo, *Charismatic leadership in organizations*, Thousand Oaks, CA: Sage, 1998, 31.

16. J. B. Engelmann, C. M. C. Capra, C. Noussair, & G. S. Berns, "Expert financial advice neurobiologically 'offloads' financial decision-making under risk," *PLoS One*, 4, e4957, quote on p. 10.

17. M. G. Edelson, Y. Dudai, R. J. Dolan, & T. Sharot, "Brain substrates of recovery from misleading influence," *Journal of Neuroscience*, 2014, 34, 7744–7753, quote on p. 7751.

18. J. A. Conger & R. N. Kanungo, *Charismatic leadership in organizations*, Thousand Oaks, CA: Sage, 1998, 63.

19. N. Nattrass, *Mortal combat: AIDS denialism and the struggle for antiretrovirals in South Africa*, KwaZulu Natal, South Africa: University of KwaZulu Natal Press, 2007, 151.

20. N. Oreskes & E. M. Conway, *Merchants of doubt*, New York: Bloomsbury Press, 2010, 10.

21. We do not mean to disparage any scientific journal and recognize that many useful and even important scientific publications find their homes in journals of lesser overall impact. However, it remains the case that there is a hierarchy of scientific and medical journals, with publications like *Science, Nature, The New*

England Journal of Medicine, and *Proceedings of the National Academy of Sciences* (PNAS) at the top. These journals conduct the most rigorous—some would say ferocious—peer review of submitted manuscripts and have very low acceptance rates, around 10% or less. As we descend the hierarchy, it gets progressively easier to get a paper accepted for publication.

22. P. H. Duesberg, *Inventing the AIDS virus,* Washington, DC: Regnery, 1998, 11.

23. R. B. Cialdini, *Influence: Science and practice,* 5th ed., Boston: Pearson Education, 2009, 212–213.

24. P. H. Duesberg, *Inventing the AIDS virus,* Washington, DC: Regnery, 1998, 66–67.

25. Two of the most disturbing aspects of this affair are that Wakefield's paper was published in the journal *Lancet,* which is considered a top-tier medical journal, and the prolonged time before the editors of *Lancet* agreed to have the paper retracted despite Wakefield's refusal to do so himself (the original paper was published in 1998 and not retracted until 2010). One can only speculate how a paper with only 12 subjects who were not properly ascertained for the study and without any comparison group possibly got past the *Lancet*'s normally rigorous review. It has since been made clear that the paper is essentially a fraud.

26. https://www.youtube.com/watch?v=l6kOxkPJfRM

27. https://www.youtube.com/watch?v=EpvB3gt4akE

28. https://www.youtube.com/watch?v=EpvB3gt4akE

29. A. Picard, "Medical fraud revealed in discredited vaccine-autism study," *The Globe and Mail,* January 6, 2011.

30. J. A. Conger & R. N. Kanungo, *Charismatic leadership in organizations,* Thousand Oaks, CA: Sage, 1998, 47.

31. J. A. Conger & R. N. Kanungo, *Charismatic leadership in organizations,* Thousand Oaks, CA: Sage, 1998, 47.

32. https://www.youtube.com/watch?v=ob1fycxZIwI

33. As will be discussed later in this book, oxytocin is a hormone secreted by a structure in the brain called the hypothalamus. Among other functions, oxytocin plays a major role in mammals in enhancing attachment behaviors, such as those between mothers and infants. When given to humans, it can make them feel more secure, loved, and affiliated with others.

34. Technically, the U.S. Department of Energy was not created until 1977, although its official website does acknowledge that it traces its lineage to the Manhattan Project, which developed the atomic bomb.

35. "Vermont v science," *The Economist*, May 10, 2014, pp. 25–26. We believe the real problem with GMOs was aptly stated by Mark Bittman in an op-ed piece in *The New York Times* on May 6, 2014: "By themselves and in their current primitive form, G.M.O.s are probably harmless; the technology itself is not even a little bit nervous making. (Neither we nor plants would be possible without 'foreign DNA' in our cells.) But to date G.M.O.s have been used by companies like Monsanto to maximize profits and further removing the accumulated expertise of generations of farmers from agriculture; in those goals, they've succeeded brilliantly. They have not been successful in moving sustainable agriculture forward (which is relevant because that was their claim), nor has their deployment been harmless: It's helped accelerate industrial agriculture and its problems and strengthened the positions of unprincipled companies. But the technology itself has not been found to be harmful." In other words, GMOs are not harmful to human health but have not been used yet to engage the problems of starvation and disease for which they could be helpful.

36. A. Harmon, "A lonely quest for facts on genetically modified crops," *The New York Times*, January 4, 2014.

37. G. E. Séralini, E. Clair, R. Mesnage, S. Gress, N. Defarge, M. Malatesta, D. Hennequin, & J. S. de Vendômois, "Long term toxicity of a Roundup herbicide and a Roundup-tolerant genetically modified maize," Food and Chemical Toxicology, 2012, 50, 4221–4231. (Note that maize is what North Americans call corn.)

38. Retraction notice to "Long term toxicity of a Roundup herbicide and a Roundup-tolerant genetically modified maize," *Food and Chemical Toxicology*, 2012, 50, 4221–4231.

39. G. E. Séralini, R. Mesnage, & N. Defarge, "Conclusiveness of toxicity data and double standards," *Food and Chemical Toxicology*, 2014, http://dx.doi.org/10.1016/j.fct2012.08.005

40. http://www.sustainablepulse.com

41. http://www.digital-athanor.com/PRISM_ESCAPE/article_usb312.html?id_article=18

42. B. Alberts, R. Beachy, D. Baulcombe, G. Blobel, S. Datta, N. Fedoroff, D. Kennedy, G. S. Khush, J. Peacock, M. Rees, & P. Sharp, "Standing up for GMOs," *Science*, 2013, *341*, 1320.

43. W. LaPierre, address to the Conservative Political Action Conference, National Harbor, Maryland, February 6, 2014, http://www.nrablog.com/post/2014/03/06/Wayne-LaPierres-address-to-the-2014-Conservative-Political-Action-Conference.aspx#continue

44. http://motleynews.net/2013/02/06/was-nra-leader-wayne-lapierre-deferred-from-vietnam-due-to-a-nervous-disorder/; https://www.facebook.com/ThePlatznerPost/posts/415418721878388; http://www.democraticunderground.com/10022302951

45. H. Stuart, "Violence and mental illness: An overview," *World Psychiatry*, 2003, *2*, 121–124.

46. C. L. Barry, E. E. McGinty, J. S. Vernick, & D. W. Webster, "After Newtown—public opinion on gun policy and mental illness," *New England Journal of Medicine*, 2013, *368*, 1077–1081.

47. http://www.nydailynews.com/news/national/nra-wayne-lapierre-tells-group-guns-protect-murderers-bloomberg-article-1.1769560

48. R. Keers, S. Ullrich, B. L. Destavola, & J. W. Coid, "Association of violence with emergence of persecutory delusions in untreated schizophrenia," *American Journal of Psychiatry*, 2014, *171*, 332–339.

49. J. W. Coil et al., "The relationship between delusions and violence: Findings from the East London First Episode Psychosis Study," *JAMA Psychiatry*, 2013, *70*, 465–471.

50. J. W. Swanson, "Explaining rare acts of violence: The limits of evidence from population research," *Psychiatry Services*, 2011, *62*, 1369–1371.

51. P. S. Appelbaum & J. W. Swanson, "Law and psychiatry: Gun laws and mental illness: How sensible are the current restrictions?" *Psychiatry Services*, 2010, *61*, 652–654.

52. American Psychiatric Association, *Fact sheet: Violence and mental illness*, Washington, DC: Author, 1994.

53. J. T. Walkup & D. H. Rubin, "Social withdrawal and violence—Newtown, Connecticut," *New England Journal of Medicine* 2013, *368*, 399–401.

54. H. Stuart, "Violence and mental illness: An overview," *World Psychiatry*, 2003, *2*, 121–124.

55. C. Mair et al., "Varying impacts of alcohol outlet densities on violent assaults: Explaining differences across neighborhoods," *Journal of Studies on Alcohol Drugs*, 2013, 74, 50.

56. G. J. Wintermute, "Association between firearm ownership, firearm-related risk and risk reduction behaviours and alcohol-related risk behaviours," *Injury Prevention*, 2011, 17, 422–427.

57. D. A. Brent, J. A. Perper, & C. J. Allman, "Alcohol, firearms, and suicide among youth," *Journal of the American Medical Association*, 1987, 257, 3369–3372; F. P. Rivara, B. A. Mueller, G. Somes, C. T. Mendoza, N. B. Rushforth, & A. L. Kellerman, "Alcohol and illicit drug abuse and the risk of violent death in the home," *Journal of the American Medical Association*, 1997, 278, 569–575.

58. "Violent, drunk and holding a gun," *The New York Times*, February 23, 2013.

59. W. LaPierre, Address to the Conservative Political Action Conference, National Harbor, Maryland, March 6, 2014, http://www.nrablog.com/post/2014/03/06/Wayne-LaPierres-address-to-the-2014-Conservative-Political-Action-Conference.aspx#continue

60. N. Oreskes & E. M. Conway, *Merchants of doubt*, New York: Bloomsbury Press, 2010, 8.

61. N. Oreskes & E. M. Conway, *Merchants of doubt*, New York: Bloomsbury Press, 2010, 27.

62. S. A. Haslam, S. D. Reicher, & M. J. Platow, *The new psychology of leadership: Identity, influence, and power*, Hove, East Sussex, UK: Psychology Press, 2011, 50.

63. S. A. Haslam, S. D. Reicher, & M. J. Platow, *The new psychology of leadership: Identity, influence, and power*, Hove, East Sussex, UK: Psychology Press, 2011, 52.

64. S. A. Haslam, S. D. Reicher, & M. J. Platow, *The new psychology of leadership: Identity, influence, and power*, Hove, East Sussex, UK: Psychology Press, 2011, 52.

65. S. A. Haslam, S. D. Reicher, & M. J. Platow, *The new psychology of leadership: Identity, influence, and power*, Hove, East Sussex, UK: Psychology Press, 2011, 55.

66. S. A. Haslam, S. D. Reicher, & M. J. Platow, *The new psychology of leadership: Identity, influence, and power*, Hove, East Sussex, UK: Psychology Press, 2011, 67–68.

67. R. H. Gass & J. S. Seiter, *Persuasion, social influence, and compliance gaining*, 4th ed., Boston: Allyn & Bacon, 2011, 117–118.

68. G. S. Berns, J. Chappelow, F. Zink, P. Pagnoni, M. E. Martin-Skurski, & J. Richards, "Neurobiological correlates of social conformity and independence during mental rotation," *Biological Psychiatry*, 2005, 58, 245–253.

69. B. G. Southwell, *Social networks and popular understanding of science and health: Sharing disparities*, Baltimore MD: The Johns Hopkins University Press, 2013, 72.

70. S. Zeki, "The neurobiology of love," *FEBS Letters*, 2007, 581, 2575–2579.

71. E. Fehr & C. F. Camerer, "Social neuroeconomics: The neural circuitry of social preferences," *Trends in Cognitive Sciences*, 2007, 11, 419–427.

72. R. H. Gass & J. S. Seiter, *Persuasion, social influence, and compliance gaining*, 4th ed., Boston: Allyn & Bacon, 2011, 120.

73. R. H. Gass & J. S. Seiter, *Persuasion, social influence, and compliance gaining*, 4th ed., Boston: Allyn & Bacon, 2011, 120.

74. Because he is a true believer that global warming is a real phenomenon that is threatening human existence, Jack affiliates with groups that share this belief and advocate for a reduction in the use of fossil fuels. However, it is often the case that such groups adopt other ideas that they think are environmentally correct, such as opposing nuclear power and GMOs. In these settings, surrounded by people he generally respects, Jack often refrains from expressing his privately held belief that neither is actually a threat. Thus, Jack in his silence and fear of being ostracized from the group, succumbs to normative influence. Fortunately, he gets to express his true feelings in this book.

75. J. A. Conger & R. N. Kanungo, *Charismatic leadership in organizations*, Thousand Oaks, CA: Sage, 1998, 272.

76. J. A. Conger & R. N. Kanungo, *Charismatic leadership in organizations*, Thousand Oaks, CA: Sage, 1998, 50.

77. D. Kelly & M. D'Aust Garcia, "Resisting persuasion: Building defences against competitors' persuasive attacks in the context of war-gaming methodology," *Journal of Medical Marketing*, 2009, 9(2), 84.

78. D. Kelly & M. D'Aust Garcia, "Resisting persuasion: Building defences against competitors' persuasive attacks in the context of war-gaming methodology," *Journal of Medical Marketing,* 2009, 9(2), 84.

79. M. Friestad & P. Wright, "The persuasion knowledge model: How people cope with persuasion attempts," *Journal of Consumer Research,* 1994, 21(1), 12.

80. J. L. Lemanski & H.-S. Lee, "Attitude certainty and resistance to persuasion: investigating the impact of source trustworthiness in advertising," *International Journal of Business and Social Science,* 2012, 3(1), 71.

81. E. S. Knowles & J. A. Linn (Eds.), Resistance and persuasion, Yahweh: Lawrence Erlbaum Associates, 2004, 29

82. N. Hertz, *Eyes wide open,* New York: HarperCollins, 2013, 70.

Chapter 3

1. For instance, the famous Yogi line "When you get to a fork in the road, take it" refers to directions he gave to get to his house, which was on a cul-de-sac. Hence, when one got to the fork in the road, going either way would serve equally well to get to his house. Yogi's statement turns out to be perfectly logical after all.

2. R. S. Nickerson, "Confirmation bias: A ubiquitous phenomenon in many guises," *Review of General Psychology,* 1998, 2, 175–220.

3. D. Alighieri, canto 13 in "Paradiso," in *The divine comedy: Inferno; purgatorio; paradiso,* trans. Allen Mandelbaum, New York: Alfred A Knopf (Everyman's Library), 1995, 441.

4. D. A. Redelmeier & A. Tversky, "On the belief that arthritis pain is related to the weather," *Proceedings of the National Academy of Medicine,* 1996, 93, 2895–2896.

5. Actually, Jack did make that mistake twice. The second umbrella was just as bad as the first. He would have been better off succumbing to confirmation bias in the first instance.

6. We often use the term "prestigious" journal. There are basically two ways that this is determined. The first is historical. Certain journals have gained reputations for being more authoritative than others over the years, and these are generally the most selective when it comes to accepting submissions. The

American journal *Science* and the British journal *Nature* are generally held as the two most prestigious scientific journals in the world. In medicine, this would be the *New England Journal of Medicine*. The second way to determine whether a journal is "prestigious" is by *impact factor*, which is a calculation based on the number of times each article in a journal is referred to, or "cited," in other scientific articles. Getting an article published in prestigious, high-impact journals is the coin of the realm for scientists, necessary for them to get tenure at their institutions, funding from granting agencies, and invitations to speak at important scientific conferences. Journalists also troll the more prestigious articles, looking for new things about which to write articles.

7. R. S. Nickerson, "Confirmation bias: A ubiquitous phenomenon in many guises," *Review of General Psychology*, 1998, 2, 175–220.

8. *Strep throat* is of course the popular phrase for infection of the mucous membrane of the throat—technically called pharyngitis—by a bacteria called streptococcus. Although most people with streptococcal pharyngitis recover uneventfully, a subgroup develop serious complications later on, including a type of kidney disease called glomerulonephritis, heart disease called rheumatic heart disease, and neurological disease called Syndenham's chorea. The first two of these can cause premature death.

9. This is the name doctors give the rash associated with *scarlet fever*, part of the complex of symptoms and signs caused by *Streptococcus*, or group A strep, infection that includes strep throat.

10. Depending on the study, only about 10% of cases of sore throat are caused by strep. The most common virus to cause pharyngitis is adenovirus, but many other viruses can do it as well.

11. This is in itself an irrational choice, since plain old penicillin is probably better than azithromycin or the Z-Pak for treating strep throat. But that is another story.

12. M. L. Barnett & J. A. Linder, "Antibiotic prescribing to adults with sore throat in the United States, 1997–2010," *JAMA Internal Medicine*, 2014, 174, 138–140. We should also note that

despite the fact that we used a pediatric example, pediatricians seem to be coming around to prescribing antibiotics for sore throats in children only when the tests are positive for strep. But changing this prescribing behavior was not easy.

13. R. M. Poses, R. D. Cebul, M. Collins, & S. S. Fager, "The accuracy of experienced physicians' probability estimates for patients with sore throats: Implications for decision making," JAMA, 1985, *254*, 925–929; M. R. Wessels, "Streptococcal pharyngitis," *New England Journal of Medicine*, 2011, *364*, 648–655.

14. M. L. Barnett & J. A. Linder, "Antibiotic prescribing for adults with acute bronchitis in the United States, 1996–2010," *JAMA*, 2014, *311*, 2020–2022.

15. It is important to note here that physicians overprescribing antibiotics contributes to the problem of creating bacterial resistance but overuse in agriculture is an even more significant factor. Antibiotics should be given only to sick livestock but are commonly given promiscuously to all farm animals. Nearly 80% of the antibiotics sold in the United States are fed to animals to promote growth, not to treat bacterial infections. The FDA has only recently started to address this serious problem, and unfortunately what they have asked for from pharmaceutical companies so far is only voluntary. The FDA does not have regulatory authority over farmers. So although we are often skeptical of claims that the food we eat is dangerous, there is no question that meat from animals treated with antibiotics is a substantial threat to our health.

16. Centers for Disease Control and Prevention (CDC), "Antibiotic/antimicrobial resistance: Threat report 2013," http://www.cdc.gov/drugresistance/threat-report-2013/index.html; "Antibiotic resistance: The spread of superbugs," *The Economist*, March 31, 2011, http://www.economist.com/node/18483671.

17. Physicians Briefing, "CDC addresses burden, threat of antibiotic resistance," www.physiciansbriefing.com/Article/asp?AID=683568, January 6, 2014.

18. "The antibiotic crisis," *The New York Times*, September 17, 2013.

19. J. P. Donnelly, J. W. Baddley, & H. E. Wang, "Antibiotic utilization for acute respiratory tract infections in U.S. emergency

departments," *Antimicrobial Agents and Chemotherapy*, 2014, 58, 1451–1457.

20. It is worth commenting here on the use of the term *cold*. The common cold is an illness caused by a group of organisms called rhinoviruses that infect that upper airways of the respiratory tract (nasal passages and throat), causing cough, sneeze, headache, fever, and general malaise. When people get sick with a cold they seem to think the word *cold* is inadequate to describe their misery. The cold is then described as a *head cold* or a *chest cold*, to distinguish what they have from an ordinary cold. These modifiers, however, have no medical significance. Colds are unpleasant and debilitating, especially in the very young, very old, or otherwise medically ill, but for most people they go away when the body's immune system is able to kill off the rhinovirus. That takes about 10 days. Antibiotics have absolutely no influence on the course of the common cold.

21. C. Llor, A. Moragas, C. Bayona, R. Morros, H. Pera, O. Plana-Ripoll, J. M. Cots, & M. Miravitlles, "Efficacy of an anti-inflammatory or antibiotic treatment in patients with non–complicated acute bronchitis and discoloured sputum: Randomised placebo controlled trial," *British Medical Journal*, 2013, 347, f5762.

22. S. Fridkin, J. Baggs, R. Fagan, et al., "Vital signs: Improving antibiotic use among hospitalized patients," http://www.cdc.gov/mmwr/preview/mmwrhtml/mm63e0304a1.htm, March 4, 2014.

23. A. Phlipson, "Britain is reaching 'a tipping point in its use of antibiotics,' says Wellcome Trust director," www.telegraph.co.uk/health/healthnews/10557959, January 8, 2014.

24. N. Teicholz, "Fat (reconsidered)," *The Wall Street Journal*, May 3–4, 2014.

25. A. Keys & F. Grande, "Role of dietary fat in human nutrition. III. Diet and the epidemiology of coronary heart disease," *American Journal of Public Health and the Nation's Health*, 1957, 47, 1520–1530. Note that Keys and Grande refer only to men when they worry about heart attacks. Back in the 1950s another mistake commonly made by physicians and the public was to believe that women don't get heart attacks. In fact, heart disease is by far the leading cause of death of women in the United States, exceeding breast cancer. Yet efforts to identify breast cancer are far more

vigorous than those to prevent unnecessary myocardial infarctions in women.

26. R. Chowdhury, S. Warnakula, S. Kunutsor, F. Crowe, H. A. Ward, L. Johnson, O. H. Franco, A. S. Butterworth, N. G. Forouhi, S. G. Thompson, K. T. Khaw, D. Mozaffarian, J. Danesh, & D. Di Angelantonio, "Association of dietary, circulating, and supplement fatty acids with coronary risk: A systematic review and meta-analysis," *Annals of Internal Medicine*, 2014, *160*, 398–406.

27. A note on meta-analysis. In this procedure, a scientist or group of scientists locates all the papers in the literature that can be found in which there are data relevant to a certain question. Then a statistical procedure is used to put all of the data together and reach a conclusion. This is especially useful in situations in which a series of studies with relatively small numbers of participants have yielded contradictory findings. By combining all the studies, a larger sample is accumulated that sometimes permits a more statistically convincing finding. There are many technical hurdles and some shortcomings to meta-analysis, but it is often useful when a subject that has been studied is still unclear.

28. Note that high cholesterol level is indeed a valid risk marker for heart attacks and this deserves intervention, with diet, exercise and/or medications called statins. It is just that how much fat you eat does not seem to be related to this process.

29. As we do note elsewhere, while the scientists who conducted these studies were *generally* acting in good faith even though their conclusions turn out to be incorrect, there is an element of conspiracy in the dietary fat recommendations. A conglomerate of food companies and medical associations worked together to make sure that the advice served their financial goals.

30. L. A. Bazzano, T. Hu, K. Reynolds, L. Yao, C. Bunol, Y. Liu, C.-S. Chen, M. J. Klag, P. K. Whelton, & J. He, "Effects of low-carbohydrate and low-fat diets," *Annals of Internal Medicine*, 2014, *161*, 309–318.

31. F. A. Goodyear-Smith, M. L. van Driel, B. Arroll, & C. H. Del Mar, "Analysis of decisions made in meta-analyses of depression screening and the risk of confirmation bias: A case study," *BMC Medical Research Methods*, 2012, *12*, 76.

32. C. A. Anderson, M. R. Lepper, & L. Ross, "Perseverance of social theories: The role of explanation in the persistence of discredited information," *Journal of Personality and Social Psychology,* 1980, *39*, 1037–1049, quote on p. 1042.

33. S. Schulz-Hardt, D. Frey, C. Lüthgens, & S. Moscovici, "Biased information search in group decision making," *Journal of Personality and Social Psychology,* 2000, *78*, 655–659.

34. It has been pointed out that the original source for this information comes from a U.K. newspaper, the *Daily Mail,* that is not necessarily reliable. However, whether or not Angelina Jolie actually said what she is quoted as saying, we are interested here in the reaction it got from gun proponents and their reaction, in turn, to Jack's challenging them with data.

35. G. Kleck & M. Gertz, "Armed resistance to crime: The prevalence and nature of self-defense with a gun," *Journal of Criminal Law and Criminology,* 1995, *86,* 150–187.

36. D. Hemenway, *Private guns, public health,* Ann Arbor: University of Michigan Press, 2004.

37. M. Shermer, "When science doesn't support our beliefs," *Scientific American,* October 2013, 95.

38. B. G. Southwell, *Social networks and popular understanding of science and health: Sharing disparities,* Baltimore: The Johns Hopkins Press, 2013, 73.

39. J. M. Boden, L. Fergusson, & J. Horwood, "Cigarette smoking and depression: Tests of causal linkages using a longitudinal birth cohort," *British Journal of Psychiatry,* 2010, *196,* 440–446.

40. In his excellent book *The Panic Virus,* Seth Mnookin discusses the isolation children of parents with autism feel and how that drives them toward participating in group causes, such as the anti-vaccine movement.

41. P. Slovic, "The affect heuristic," in T. Bilovich, D. Griffin, & D. Kahneman, eds., *Heuristics and biases: The psychology of intuitive judgment,* New York: Cambridge University Press, 2002, 401.

42. P. Slovic, "The affect heuristic," in T. Bilovich, D. Griffin, & D. Kahneman, eds., *Heuristics and biases: The psychology of intuitive judgment,* New York: Cambridge University Press, 2002, 410.

43. N. Schwarz, "Feelings as information: Moods influence judgments and processing strategies," in T. Bilovich, D. Griffin, & D.

Kahneman, eds., *Heuristics and biases: The psychology of intuitive judgment*, New York: Cambridge University Press, 2002.

44. B. G. Southwell, *Social networks and popular understanding of science and health: Sharing disparities*, Baltimore: The Johns Hopkins Press, 2013, 97.

45. G. S. Berns, J. Chappelow, C. F. Zink, G. Pagnoni, M. E. Martin-Skurski, & J. Richards, "Neurobiological correlates of social conformity and independence during mental rotation," *Biological Psychiatry*, 2005, *58*, 245–253.

46. E. G. Falk & M. D. Lieberman, "The neural bases of attitudes, evaluation, and behavior change," in F. Krueger & J. Grafman, eds., *The neural basis of human belief systems*, Hove, East Sussex, UK: Psychology Press, 2013.

47. S. A. Sloman, "Two systems of reasoning," in T. Bilovich, D. Griffin, & D. Kahneman, eds., *Heuristics and biases: The psychology of intuitive judgment*, New York: Cambridge University Press, 2002.

48. This statement will not go unchallenged, and indeed research is increasingly suggesting that other species demonstrate altruism. Suffice it to say here, however, that if chimpanzees and other great apes are really capable of charitable behavior for its own sake it is much harder to recognize than such behavior in humans.

49. K. E. Stanovich & R. F. West, "On the failure of cognitive ability to predict myside and one-sided thinking biases," *Thinking and Reasoning*, 2008, *14*, 129–167; K. E. Stanovich, R. F. West, & M. E. Toplak, "Myside bias, rationale thinking, and intelligence," *Current Direction in Psychological Science*, 2013, *22*, 259–264.

50. C. M. Kuhnen & B. Knutson, "The neural basis of financial risk," *Neuron*, 2005, *47*, 763–770.

51. N. Hertz, *Eyes wide open*, New York: HarperCollins, 2013, 38.

52. C. M. Kuhnen & J. Y. Chiao, "Genetic determinants of financial risk taking," *PLoS One*, 2009, *4*, e4362.

53. C. M. Kuhnen, G. R. Samanez-Larkin, & B. Knutson, "Serotonergic genotypes, neuroticism, and financial choices," *PLoS One*, 2013, *8*, e54632.

54. C. G. Lord, L. Ross, & M. R. Lepper, "Biased assimilation and attitude polarization: The effects of prior theories on subsequently considered evidence," *Journal of Personality and Social Psychology*, 1979, 37, 2098–2109, quote on p. 2098.
55. A. T. Beck, *Cognitive therapy and the emotional disorders*, New York: International Universities Press, 1976.
56. C. A. Anderson, M. R. Lepper, & L. Ross, "Perseverance of social theories: The role of explanation in the persistence of discredited information," *Journal of Personality and Social Psychology*, 1980, 39, 1037–1049, quote on p. 1048.
57. L. Rosenbaum, "'Misrearing'—culture, identify, and our perceptions of health risks," *New England Journal of Medicine*, 2014, 37, 595–597, quote on p. 597.

Chapter 4

1. http://plato.stanford.edu/entries/causation-counterfactual/
2. It is surprising to learn that only a minority of people who regularly smoke actually develop adenocarcinoma of the lung. But this should not be taken as comforting news. First, people who don't smoke almost never get lung cancer, so the difference is staggering. Second, lung cancer is only one of a host of cancers and other devastating diseases that smoking causes. Most smokers sooner or later get a disease related to smoking, even if it isn't lung cancer. At the present time, the Surgeon General officially lists 21 different diseases caused by cigarette smoking and there is now compelling evidence that there are even more.
3. S. A. Vyse, *Believing in magic: The psychology of superstition*, rev. ed., Oxford: Oxford University Press, 2000, 74.
4. S. A. Vyse, *Believing in magic: The psychology of superstition*, rev. ed., Oxford: Oxford University Press, 2000, 76.
5. S. A. Vyse, *Believing in magic: The psychology of superstition*, rev. ed., Oxford: Oxford University Press, 2000, 74.
6. R. Park, *Voodoo science: The road from foolishness to fraud*, Oxford: Oxford University Press, 2000, 35–36.
7. In fact, this is often a case of association, not causality. Many people without back pain have herniated discs, so it is not always clear that finding one on an MRI explains the cause of

pain. See, for example, M. C. Jensen, M. N. Brant-Zawadzki, N. Obuchowski, M. T. Modic, D. Malkasian, & J. S. Ross, "Magnetic resonance imaging of the lumbar spine in people without back pain," *New England Journal of Medicine*, 1994, 331, 69–73.

8. D. Ariely, *Predictably irrational: The hidden forces that shape our decisions*, New York: Harper Perennial, 2009.

9. T. Kida, *Don't believe everything you think: The 6 basic mistakes we make in thinking*, Amherst, NY: Prometheus Books, 2006, 86.

10. M. Shermer, *Why people believe weird things: Pseudoscience, superstition, and other confusions of our time*, New York: St. Martin's Griffin, 2002, 59.

11. M. E. Talkowski, E. V. Minikel, & J. F. Gusellam, "Autism spectrum disorder genetics: Diverse genes with diverse clinical outcomes," *Harvard Review of Psychiatry*, 2015, 22, 65–75; S. Sandin, D. Schendel, P. Magnusson, et al., "Autism risk associated with parental age and with increasing difference in age between the parents," *Molecular Psychiatry*, 2015, doi:10.1038/mp.2015.70, Epub ahead of print.

12. K. R. Foster & H. Kokko, "The evolution of superstitious and superstition-like behavior," *Proceedings of the Royal Society of Biological Sciences*, 2009, 276, 31.

13. K. R. Foster & H. Kokko, "The evolution of superstitious and superstition-like behavior," *Proceedings of the Royal Society of Biological Sciences*, 2009, 276, 31.

14. S. A. Vyse, *Believing in magic: The psychology of superstition*, rev. ed., Oxford: Oxford University Press, 2000, 86.

15. http://www.forbes.com/2009/03/06/superstitious-ufo-alien-conspiracy-opinions-columnists-superstition.html

16. A. Bandura, D. Ross, & S. A. Ross, "Transmission of aggression through the imitation of aggressive models," *Journal of Abnormal and Social Psychology*, 1961, 63 (3): 575–582.

17. L. Damisch, B. Stoberock, & T. Mussweiler, "Keep your fingers crossed! How superstition improves performance," *Psychological Science*, 2010, 21, 1014–1020. Experts in polling may question our wisdom in citing such a Gallup poll but we will give them the benefit of the doubt this time.

18. S. A. Vyse, *Believing in magic: The psychology of superstition*, rev. ed., Oxford: Oxford University Press, 2000, 118; T. Kida,

Don't believe everything you think: The 6 basic mistakes we make in thinking, Amherst, NY: Prometheus Books, 2006, 92.

19. S. A. Vyse, *Believing in magic: The psychology of superstition*, rev. ed., Oxford: Oxford University Press, 2000, 140.
20. S. A. Vyse, *Believing in magic: The psychology of superstition*, rev. ed., Oxford: Oxford University Press, 2000, 140.

Chapter 5

1. *New York Daily News*, Tuesday, April 22, 2014.
2. F. Bruni, "Autism and the agitator," *The New York Times*, Tuesday, April 22, 2014. Also, don't get us started on the issue of gluten-free diets, another major boondoggle of the health food industry. There is a well-characterized medical condition called celiac disease in which the patient makes antibodies to a protein in wheat called gluten that cross-react against cells of the intestinal lining or mucosa, causing horrible inflammation and damage up and down the small intestine. These individuals become malnourished and very ill unless they eliminate gluten from their diets. The disease can now be readily diagnosed by a blood test that identifies antibodies called antitissue transglutaminase antibodies (tTGA) or anti-endomysial antibodies (EMA). It turns out that the vast majority of people who think they have some kind of gluten sensitivity actually do not. It is important to remember that whereas humans have about 20,000 to 30,000 genes and two sets of chromosomes, wheat has about 90,000 genes and as many as six sets of chromosomes. So it may be the case that some people with GI problems are abnormally sensitive to wheat, but unless they have celiac disease it isn't to gluten, and eating a gluten-free diet is useless. It could, however, be one of the other 89,999 proteins expressed by the wheat genome.
3. D. M. Kahan, "A risky science communication environment for vaccines," *Science*, 2013, 342, 53–54.
4. This notion does seem a bit silly. There is no evidence that teenagers currently *refrain* from having sex because of fear of becoming infected with HPV or getting cervical cancer, so exactly how a vaccine against HPV would increase sexual activity in adolescents remains a mystery.
5. J. LeDoux, *The emotional brain*, New York: Touchstone, 1996.

6. F. Krueger & J. Grafman, *The neural basis of human belief systems*, East Sussex, UK: Psychology Press, 2013, xii.

7. A. Shenhav & J. D. Greene, "Integrative moral judgment: Dissociating the roles of the amygdala and ventromedial prefrontal cortex," *The Journal of Neuroscience*, 2014, *34*, 4741–4749.

8. S. M. McClure, D. I. Laibson, G. Loewenstein, & J. D. Cohen, "Separate neural systems value immediate and delayed monetary rewards," *Science*, 2004, *306*, 503–507.

9. E. B. Falk & M. D. Lieberman, "The neural bases of attitudes, evaluation, and behavior change," in F. Krueger & J. Grafman, eds., *The neural basis of human belief systems*, East Sussex, UK: Psychology Press, 2013, 85.

10. D. Kahneman, *Thinking, fast and slow*, New York: Farrar, Straus and Geroux, 2011, 98.

11. R. H. Thaler & C. R. Sunstein, *Nudge: Improving decisions about health, wealth, and happiness*, London: Penguin Books, 2008.

12. H. P. Spaans, P. Seinaert, F. Boukaert, J. F. van den Berg, E. Verwijk, K. H. Kho, M. L. Stek, & R. M. Kok, "Speed of remission in elderly patients with depression: Electroconvulsive therapy v. medication," *British Journal of Psychiatry*, 2015, *206*, 67–71.

13. S, Sloman, "The empirical case for two systems of reasoning," *Psychological Bulletin*, 1996, *119*, 3–22.

14. Pew Research Center for the People and the Press "Public's knowledge of science and technology," http://www.people-press.org/2013/04/22/publics-knowledge-of-science-and-technology/, accessed April 11, 2014.

15. J. D. Miller, "The public understanding of science in Europe and the United States," paper presented at the AAAS annual meeting, San Francisco, CA, February 16, 2007, as reported in Janet Raloff, "Science literacy: U.S. college courses really count," https://www.sciencenews.org/blog/science/public/science-literacy-us-college-courses-really-count, accessed April 1, 2014.

16. J. Mervis, "Why many U.S. biology teachers are 'wishy-washy,'" *Science*, 2015, *347*, 1054–1053.

17. L. Rainie, "Despite esteem for science, public at odds with scientists on major issues [guest blog]," *Scientific American,* http://blogs.scientificamerican.com/guest-blog/despite-esteem-for-science-public-at-odds-with-scientists-on-major-issues/, January 29, 2015.

18. J. Tanenbaum, "Creation, evolution and indisputable facts," *Scientific American,* 2013, *308,* 11.

19. J. Cohen, "Things I have learned (so far)," *American Psychologist,* 1990, *45*(12), 1304–1312.

20. F. Campbell, G. Counti, J. J. Heckman, S. Y. Moon, R. Pinto, E. Pungello, & Y. Pan, "Early childhood investments substantially boost adult health," *Science,* 2014, *343,* 1478–1485.

21. A very interesting and potentially useful approach to educating the public about how science works and how to understand scientific claims can be found in W. J. Sutherland, D. Spiegelhalter, & M. Burgman, "Policy: Twenty tips for interpreting scientific claims," *Nature,* November 20, 2013, www.nature.com/news/policy-twenty-tips-for-interpreting-scientific-claims-1.14183?WT.mc_id=FBK_NatureNews

22. S. Kirshenbaum, "No, the sun does not revolve around the Earth," http://www.cnn.com/2014/02/18/opinion/kirshenbaum-science-literacy/index.html, accessed April 1, 2014.

23. R. J. DeRubeis, G. J. Siegle, & S. D. Hollon, "Cognitive therapy versus medication for depression: Treatment outcomes and neural mechanisms," *Nature Reviews Neuroscience,* 2008, *9,* 788–796.

24. R. Yu, D. Mobbs, B. Seymour, & A. J. Calder, "Insula and striatum mediate the default bias," *Journal of Neuroscience,* 2010, *30,* 14702–14707.

25. K. M. Harlé, L. J. Chang, M. van 't Wout, & A. G. Sanfey, "The neural mechanisms of affect infusion in social economic decision-making: A mediating role of the anterior insula," *Neuroimage,* 2012, *61,* 32–40.

26. M. Browning, T. E. Behrens, G. Jocham, J. X. O'Reilly, & S. J. Bishop, "Anxious individuals have difficulty learning the causal statistics of aversive environments," *Nature Neuroscience,* 2015, *18,* 590–596.

27. S. Wang, "How to think about the risk of autism," *The New York Times*, March 29, 2014, http://www.nytimes.com/2014/03/30/opinion/sunday/how-to-think-about-the-risk-of-autism.html

28. E. B. Falk & M. D. Lieberman, "The neural bases of attitudes, evaluation, and behavior change," in F. Krueger & J. Grafman, eds., *The neural basis of human belief systems*, East Sussex, UK: Psychology Press, 2013, 76.

29. For an entertaining tour de force of similar correlations of specious meaning, see Tyler Vigen's wonderful book *Spurious Correlations*, New York: Hachette Books, 2015. You will learn that there are actually statistically significant correlations between such things as consumption of fats and oils and households that still have a VCR; U.S. citizens who are able to receive a text message and the price to send a letter via the U.S. Postal Service; and physical retail sales of video games and UFO sighting in Massachusetts. These correlations are really mathematical artifacts and can best be characterized as coincidences. But, as Casey Stengel would have said, you can't make this stuff up.

30. C. Saint Louis, "Most doctors give in to requests by parents to alter vaccine schedules," *The New York Times*, March 2, 2015, http://nyti.ms/1E8yhRZ

Chapter 6

1. http://www.cdc.gov/mmwr/preview/mmwrhtml/mm6022a1.htm. Incidentally, if you are wondering about the coin-flip rule, it is useful to point out that this is one of those "What question are you asking?" situations. The analogy to the risk of failing in the showering isn't the question "What are your odds of tossing a head (or tail) on each toss?" but rather "What are the odds of tossing at least one head (or one tail) if we toss the coin, say, 1,000 times?" The answer is well over 99%.

2. http://www.census.gov/compendia/statab/2012/tables/12s1103.pdf

3. http://www.cdc.gov/vaccines/vac-gen/6mishome.htm#risk

4. http://www.nytimes.com/2010/03/09/health/research/09child.html?_r=0

5. http://arstechnica.com/science/2012/08/widespread-vaccine-exemptions-are-messing-with-herd-immunity/

6. http://contemporarypediatrics.modernmedicine.com/contemporary-pediatrics/news/modernmedicine/modern-medicine-now/declining-vaccination-rates

7. http://www.bbc.co.uk/news/health-22277186

8. P. Narang, A. Paladugu, S. R. Manda, W. Smock, C. Gosnay, & S. Lippman, "Do guns provide safety? At what cost?" *Southern Medical Journal*, 2010, *103*, 151–153.

9. D. J. Wiebe, "Homicide and suicide risks associated with firearms in the home: A national case-controlled study," *Annals of Emergency Medicine*, 2003, *41*, 771–782.

10. C. C. Branas, T. S. Richmond, D. P. Culhane, T. R. Ten Have, & D. J. Wiebe, "Investigating the link between gun possession and gun assault," *American Journal of Public Health*, 2009, *99*, 2034–2040.

11. D. Hemenway, *Private guns, public health*, Ann Arbor: University of Michigan Press, 2004, 111.

12. A. L. Kellermann & J. A. Mercy, "Men, women, and murder: Gender-specific differences in rates of fatal violence and victimization," *Journal of Trauma*, 1992, *33*, 1–5.

13. American Academy of Pediatrics, "Firearm-related injuries affecting the pediatric population," *Pediatrics*, 2012, *130*, e1416–e1423.

14. http://www.gallup.com/poll/1645/guns.aspx

15. http://blogs.scientificamerican.com/observations/most-people-say-they-are-safe-drivers-want-new-auto-assist-tech-anyway/. An average is what statisticians call a mean and is calculated by dividing the total value of all observations by the total number of observations. If we had a rating scale for driving skill that ranged from 1 to 10, some drivers would score 1 (keep them off the road) and some 10 (nearly perfect). To get the mean or average, we would add up the total scores of all the drivers in a sample and then divide by the number of drivers in the sample. If the scores were "normally" distributed (i.e., forming a bell-shaped curve), then the average score would be 5 and half of the people would be "better than average" and half worse than average. If you do the arithmetic here, you will

find that it is virtually impossible to imagine any sample in which 90% of the drivers are better than average.

16. D. Kahneman, *Thinking, fast and slow*, New York: Farrar, Straus and Giroux, 2011, 98.

17. http://www.ncbi.nlm.nih.gov/pubmed/3563507

18. A. Markandya & P. Wilkinson, "Electricity generation and health," *Lancet*, 2007, *370*(9591), 979–990.

19. W. R. Stauffer, A. Lak, P. Bossaerts, & W. Schultz, "Economic choices reveal probability distortion in Macaque monkeys," *Journal of Neuroscience*, 2015, *35*, 3146–31534.

20. M. Hsu, I. Krajbich, C. Zhao, & C. F. Camerer, "Neural response to reward anticipation under risk is nonlinear in probabilities," *Journal of Neuroscience*, 2009, *29*, 2231–2237.

21. B. Fischhoff, S. Lichtenstein, P. Slovic, S. L. Derby, & R. L. Keeney, *Acceptable risk*, Cambridge: Cambridge University Press, 1981, 7.

22. B. Fischhoff, S. Lichtenstein, P. Slovic, S. L. Derby, & R. L. Keeney, *Acceptable risk*, Cambridge: Cambridge University Press, 1981, 15.

23. R. E. Kasperson, O. Renn, P. Slovic, H. S. Brown, J. Emel, et al., "The social amplification of risk: A conceptual framework," *Risk Analysis*, 1988, *8*(2), 184.

24. R. E. Kasperson, O. Renn, P. Slovic, H. S. Brown, J. Emel, et al., "The social amplification of risk: A conceptual framework," *Risk Analysis*, 1988, *8*(2), 184.

25. We acknowledge that there are of course other objections to nuclear power, most important of which is the issue of what to do with nuclear waste products. While we believe that this is a tractable problem and that nuclear power is still a preferable source of energy, we will not deal here with anything other than health issues. Of course, there are forms of energy that are probably even safer than nuclear, like solar and wind power, but it is unclear how easy it will be harness them to the scale needed in time to save Earth from its impending meltdown.

26. http://www.ucsusa.org/nuclear-power/nuclear-power-and-global-warming#.VvQHqhIrJBx

27. B. J. McNeil, S. G. Pauker, H. C. SoxJr., & A. Tversky, "On the elicitation of preference for alternative therapies," *New England Journal of Medicine*, 1982, *306*, 1259–1262.

28. P. Slovic, H. Kunreuther, & G. White, "Decision processes, rationality and adjustment to natural hazards," in P. Slovic, ed., *The perception of risk*, London: Earthscan, 2000, 1–31, 13.

29. T. Kida, *Don't believe everything you think: The 6 basic mistakes we make in thinking*, Amherst, NY: Prometheus Books, 2006, 174–175.

30. T. Kida, *Don't believe everything you think: The 6 basic mistakes we make in thinking*, Amherst, NY: Prometheus Books, 2006, 175.

31. D Kahneman, *Thinking, fast and slow*, New York: Farrar, Straus and Giroux, 2011, 249.

32. http://blogs.scientificamerican.com/guest-blog/2011/01/06/in-the-wake-of-wakefield-risk-perception-and-vaccines/

33. http://www.unc.edu/~ntbrewer/pubs/2007,%20brewer,%20chpaman,%20gibbons,%20et%20al.pdf

34. M. Olpinski, "Anti-vaccination movement and parental refusals of immunization of children in USA," *Pediatria Polska*, 2012, *87*, 382.

35. G. A. Poland & R. M. Jacobson, "Understanding those who do not understand: A brief review of the anti-vaccine movement," *Vaccine*, 2001, *19*, 2442.

36. M. L. Finucane, A. Alhakami, P. Slovic, & S. M Johnson, "The affect heuristic in judgments of risks and benefits," in P. Slovic, ed., *The perception of risk*, London: Earthscan, 2000, 413–429, 415–416.

37. B. Baldur-Felskov, C. Dehlendorff, J. Junge, C. Munk, & S. K. Kjaer, "Incidence of cervical lesions in Danish women before and after implementation of a national HPV vaccination program," *Cancer Causes & Control*, 2014, *25*, 915–922; D. M. Gertig, J. M. Brotherton, A. C. Budd, K. Drennan, G. Chappell, & A. M. Saville, "Impact of a population-based HPV vaccination program on cervical abnormalities: A data linkage study," *BMC Medicine*, 2013, *11*, 227.

38. M. H. Repacholi, A. Lerchl, M. Röösli, et al., "Systematic review of wireless phone use and brain cancer and other head tumors," *Bioelectromagnetics*, 2012, *33*, 187–206.

39. L. Hardell & M. Carlberg, "Mobile phone and cordless phone use and the risk for glioma—Analysis of pooled case-control studies

in Sweden, 1997–2003 and 2007–2009," *Pathophysiology*, 2015, 22, 1–13.

40. D. Kahneman, J. L. Knetsch, & R. H. Thaler, "Anomalies: The endowment effect, loss aversion, and status quo bias," *The Journal of Economic Perspectives*, 1991, 5(1), 194.

41. D. Kahneman, J. L. Knetsch, & R. H. Thaler, "Anomalies: The endowment effect, loss aversion, and status quo bias," *The Journal of Economic Perspectives*, 1991, 5(1), 195.

42. B. Knutson, G. E. Wimmer, S. Rick, N. G. Hollon, D. Prelec, & G. Loewenstein, "Neural antecedents of the endowment effect," *Neuron*, 2008, 58, 814–822.

43. D. Kahneman, J. L. Knetsch, & R. H. Thaler, "Anomalies: The endowment effect, loss aversion, and status quo bias," *The Journal of Economic Perspectives*, 1991, 5(1), 205.

44. N. Schwarz, "Feelings as information: Moods influence judgments and processing strategies," in T. Gilovich, D. W. Griffin, & D. Kahneman, eds., *Heuristics and biases*, New York: Cambridge University Press, 2002.

45. N. Schwarz, "Feelings as information: Moods influence judgments and processing strategies," in T. Gilovich, D. W. Griffin, & D. Kahneman, eds., *Heuristics and biases*, New York: Cambridge University Press, 2002, 545.

46. D. A. Eckles & B. F. Schaffner, "Loss aversion and the framing of the health care reform debate," *The Forum*, 2010, 8(1), 2.

47. D. A. Eckles & B. F. Schaffner, "Loss aversion and the framing of the health care reform debate," *The Forum*, 2010, 8(1), 4.

48. R. D. Bartels, K. M. Kelly & A. J. Rothman, "Moving beyond the function of the health behavior: The effect of message frame on behavioural decision-making," *Psychology and Health*, 2010, 25, 821–838. Incidentally, there is actually no such vaccine.

49. P. Slovic, "Informing and educating the public about risk," in P. Slovic, ed., *The perception of risk*, London: Earthscan, 2000, 185.

50. P. Slovic, "Informing and educating the public about risk," in P. Slovic, ed., *The perception of risk*, London: Earthscan, 2000, 185, 200.

51. R. H. Gass & J. S. Seiter, *Persuasion, social influence, and compliance gaining*, 4th ed., Boston: Allyn & Bacon, 2011, 135.

52. R. H. Gass & J. S. Seiter, *Persuasion, social influence, and compliance gaining*, 4th ed., Boston: Allyn & Bacon, 2011, 135.

53. C. W. Scherer and H. Cho, "A social network contagion theory of risk perception," *Risk Analysis*, 2003, 23(2), 266.

54. R. E. Kasperson, O. Renn, P. Slovic, H. S. Brown, J. Emel, et al., "The social amplification of risk: A conceptual framework," *Risk Analysis*, 1988, 8(2), 178–179.

55. R. E. Kasperson, O. Renn, P. Slovic, H. S. Brown, J. Emel, et al., "The social amplification of risk: A conceptual framework," *Risk Analysis*, 1988, 8(2), 177–178.

56. R. E. Kasperson, O. Renn, P. Slovic, H. S. Brown, J. Emel, et al., "The social amplification of risk: A conceptual framework," *Risk Analysis*, 1988, 8(2), 181.

57. http://vactruth.com/news/

58. http://www.vaccinationdebate.net/articles.html

Conclusion

1. http://www.forbes.com/sites/robertpearl/2014/03/20/a-doctors-take-on-the-anti-vaccine-movement/

2. G. A. Poland & R. M. Jacobson, "Understanding those who do not understand: a brief review of the anti-vaccine movement," *Vaccine*, 2001, 19(17–19), 2440–5.

3. http://www.cdnsciencepub.com/blog/scientific-societies-in-the-internet-age.aspx

4. M. McCartney, "Making sure that inquiry is elementary," *Science*, 2015, 348, 151–152.

5. D. Kahneman, personal communication by email, May 7, 2014.

About the Authors

Sara E. Gorman, PhD, MPH, is a public health specialist at a large multinational healthcare company, where she works on global mental health, increasing the quality of evidence in the global health field, and alternative funding models for global health. She has written extensively about global health, HIV/AIDS policy, and women's health, among other topics, for a variety of health and medical journals, including *PLoS Medicine, International Journal of Women's Health,* and *AIDS Care*. She has worked in the policy division at the HIV Law Project and as a researcher at the Epidemiology Department at Harvard School of Public Health. Dr. Gorman received her B.A. from the University of Pennsylvania, Masters of Public Health from Columbia University Mailman School of Public Health, and her PhD in English literature from Harvard University.

Jack M. Gorman, MD, is CEO and Chief Scientific Officer of Franklin Behavioral Health Consultants. Dr. Gorman was on the faculty of Columbia University's Department of Psychiatry for 25 years, eventually serving as Lieber Professor of Psychiatry. He then became the Esther and Joseph Klingenstein Professor and Chair of Psychiatry and Professor of Neuroscience at the Mount Sinai School of Medicine. He has authored or coauthored more than 400 scientific publications and was continuously funded for his research by the National Institutes of Health for 25 years. Dr. Gorman is coeditor of two Oxford University Press textbooks, *A Guide to Treatments That Work,* now in its fourth edition, and the *Comprehensive Textbook of AIDS Psychiatry,* second edition in preparation. He is author of the popular book *The Essential Guide to Psychiatric Drugs,* which appeared in its fourth edition in 2007. Dr. Gorman received his B.A. from the University of Pennsylvania and his M.D. from the College of Physicians and Surgeons of Columbia University.

Index

References to figures and tables are denoted by an italicized *f* and *t*